AF690276

Technology and Global Public Health: Volume I

Technology and Global Public Health: Volume I

Bruce Johnson

AMERICAN
MEDICAL PUBLISHERS
www.americanmedicalpublishers.com

AMERICAN
MEDICAL PUBLISHERS
www.americanmedicalpublishers.com

Cataloging-in-publication Data

Technology and global public health : volume I / Bruce Johnson.
p. cm.
Includes bibliographical references and index.
ISBN 979-8-88740-486-8
1. Medical technology. 2. World health. 3. Public health.
4. Medical innovations. I. Johnson, Bruce.
R855.3 .T43 2023
610.285--dc23

© American Medical Publishers, 2023

American Medical Publishers,
41 Flatbush Avenue,
1st Floor, New York,
NY 11217, USA

ISBN 979-8-88740-486-8 (Hardback)

This book contains information obtained from authentic and highly regarded sources. All chapters are published with permission under the Creative Commons Attribution Share Alike License or equivalent. A wide variety of references are listed. Permissions and sources are indicated; for detailed attributions, please refer to the permissions page. Reasonable efforts have been made to publish reliable data and information, but the authors, editors and publisher cannot assume any responsibility for the validity of all materials or the consequences of their use.

Trademark Notice: Registered trademark of products or corporate names are used only for explanation and identification without intent to infringe.

Contents

Preface VII

Part 1 **Healthcare and the Creation of a Data Science Ecosystem** 1

Chapter 1 **Role of HIT in Healthcare Systems and Data Science** 3
Louis Agha-Mir-Salim and Raymond Francis Sarmiento

Chapter 2 **Role of Design Thinking in Solving Challenges Related to Frail Elderly People** 16
Tony Gallanis

Chapter 3 **Developing Product Innovation in LMICs** 33
Christopher Moses

Chapter 4 **EHR Databases: Development and Use** 53
Lucas Bulgarelli, Antonio Núñez-Reiz and Rodrigo Octavio Deliberato

Chapter 5 **Global Health Projects and Financial Resources** 63
Katharine Morley, Michael Morley and Andrea Beratarrechea

Chapter 6 **System Dynamics Models and CLDs** 73
Gary Lin, Michele Palopoli and Viva Dadwal

Chapter 7 **Digital Health and the Usage of Blockchain** 94
Philip Christian C. Zuniga, Rose Ann C. Zuniga, Marie Jo-anne Mendoza, Ada Angeli Cariaga, Raymond Francis Sarmiento and Alvin B. Marcelo

Part 2 **Applications of Data Science in Healthcare** 103

Chapter 8 **Statistical Methods and their Usage in Python** 105
Calvin J. Chiew

Chapter 9 **Machine Learning for Phenotyping: Data Preparation and Analysis** 122
Cátia M. Salgado and Susana M. Vieira

Chapter 10 **Machine Learning for Phenotyping: Clustering and Unsupervised Learning** 143
Cátia M. Salgado and Susana M. Vieira

Chapter 11 **Machine Learning for Phenotyping: Learning Under Supervision** 161
Cátia M. Salgado and Susana M. Vieira

Chapter 12 **Machine Learning Techniques and their Application in Clinical Prediction Tasks** **190**
Wei-Hung Weng

Chapter 13 **Modeling and Prediction Tools: Random Forest and Support Vector Machines** **209**
Siqi Liu, Hao Du and Mengling Feng

Permissions

Index

Preface

Health is a state of complete physical, mental, and social well-being with the absence of disease and infirmity. It can be improved by encouraging healthy behaviors such as regular physical activity, appropriate sleep, as well as reducing or avoiding unhealthy behaviors or situations, such as smoking or excessive stress. In the context of public health, it is the science of preventing disease, prolonging life, and promoting health via organized efforts and informed choices of society. At the global level, it is the field of study, research, and practice that focuses on improving health and establishing health equity for all people around the world. In order to meet the health requirements of public, it is important to adapt various technological innovations in the field on global public health. This book explores all the important aspects of technology and its role in global public health in the present day scenario. A number of latest researches have been included to keep the readers up-to-date with the upcoming concepts in this area of study.

This book is a result of research of several months to collate the most relevant data in the field.

When I was approached with the idea of this book and the proposal to edit it, I was overwhelmed. It gave me an opportunity to reach out to all those who share a common interest with me in this field. I had 3 main parameters for editing this text:

1. Accuracy - The data and information provided in this book should be up-to-date and valuable to the readers.

2. Structure - The data must be presented in a structured format for easy understanding and better grasping of the readers.

3. Universal Approach - This book not only targets students but also experts and innovators in the field, thus my aim was to present topics which are of use to all.

Thus, it took me a couple of months to finish the editing of this book.

I would like to make a special mention of my publisher who considered me worthy of this opportunity and also supported me throughout the editing process. I would also like to thank the editing team at the back-end who extended their help whenever required.

Bruce Johnson

Part I
Healthcare and the Creation of a Data Science Ecosystem

1

Role of HIT in Healthcare Systems and Data Science

Louis Agha-Mir-Salim and Raymond Francis Sarmiento

Abstract *Background* Healthcare systems function as an important component and a contributing factor in global health. The application of information technology (IT) in healthcare systems function as a basis for the utilization of data science, which—in its practical application—not only provides opportunities to increase the quality of care, improve efficiency, and decrease costs but also buries the risk of hindering existing workflows, decreasing staff satisfaction, and further siloing access to patient data. *Methods* Three different applications of health information technology (HIT), applied in the context of data science, will be examined in this chapter with regard to their opportunities and challenges for the system and, as a result of this, for global health. *Results* Electronic health records, health information exchange, and artificial intelligence have great potential to alleviate some of healthcare systems' greatest burdens and make modern medicine more evidence-based, yet their successful implementation yields a multidisciplinary approach, constant development and evaluation, and collaboration amongst all stakeholders. *Conclusions* Stakeholders and implementers must consider the opportunities and challenges that come with the planning, implementation, and maintenance of HIT in order to minimize negative impacts and leverage its full potential for an overall improvement of global health.

Keywords Health information technology · Electronic health records · Health information exchange · Artificial intelligence (AI)

Learning Objectives

In this chapter, we discuss the role of health information technology (HIT) in increasingly complex, challenging, and constantly evolving healthcare systems with regard to its role in data science (*for more details on the methods of data science, please refer*

L. Agha-Mir-Salim (✉)
Faculty of Medicine, University of Southampton, Southampton, UK
e-mail: mirsalim@mit.edu

Laboratory for Computational Physiology, Massachusetts Institute of Technology, Cambridge, MA, USA

R. F. Sarmiento
University of the Philippines Manila, Manila, Philippines

to subsequent chapters of this book). We focus on how modern technologies, such as electronic health records, health information exchange, and artificial intelligence, find application in healthcare systems and how this, in turn, provides opportunities to leverage data for improvement of care quality and efficiency. We also approach the difficulties and unintended consequences that arise from the adoption and integration of such technologies into existing healthcare systems and their workflows. Besides considering technical barriers, we also examine the human layer as an important component of driving change within this domain. Finally, we will draw conclusions on where HIT is adding value for purposes of data science and provide recommendations where barriers yet need to be overcome in maximizing their potential to enhance healthcare as a highly complex component of global health.

1.1 Background

Although not explicitly mentioned in definitions of global health, healthcare systems can be viewed as an instrument or executive tool that governments and organizations deploy in striving for global health. With one of its core aspects comprising "both [the] prevention in populations and clinical care of individuals" (Koplan et al. 2009), global health is very much is reliant on healthcare systems as a subordinate framework to achieve its set goals.

Nevertheless, healthcare in itself is a highly complex and information-intensive field. The increasing integration of technology has allowed healthcare decision-makers to collect, process, and analyze this data for a more effective care delivery while enhancing the safety of patients and consumers (Singh and Sittig 2016). Considering the newly gained abundance of all health data—collected through health information technology (HIT)—coupled with the drastic developments in the field of data science (*for more details on the methods of data science, please refer to subsequent chapters of this book*) over the last decade, allows us to reimagine the practice of healthcare with evermore applications to address the industry's dynamic challenges of improving care quality, decreasing costs, guaranteeing equitable access, and fostering public health surveillance; all key components of achieving Universal Health Coverage (World Health Organization 2013).

In efforts to improve healthcare through digitization, varying approaches within and between countries have been taken, including the introduction of electronic health records (EHRs), telehealth and telemedicine, electronic learning and decision support systems, mobile health (mHealth) applications, real-time surveillance systems, artificial intelligence, etc. (Figure 1.1) (World Health Organization 2016). eHealth, often used interchangeably with HIT, is defined as the "the cost-effective and secure use of information and communications technologies (ICT) in support of health and health-related fields, including health-care services, health surveillance, health literature, and health education, knowledge and research" (World Health Assembly 2005, p. 121). It facilitates countries' health agenda by improving operational processes of service delivery, building workforce capacity, and engaging all

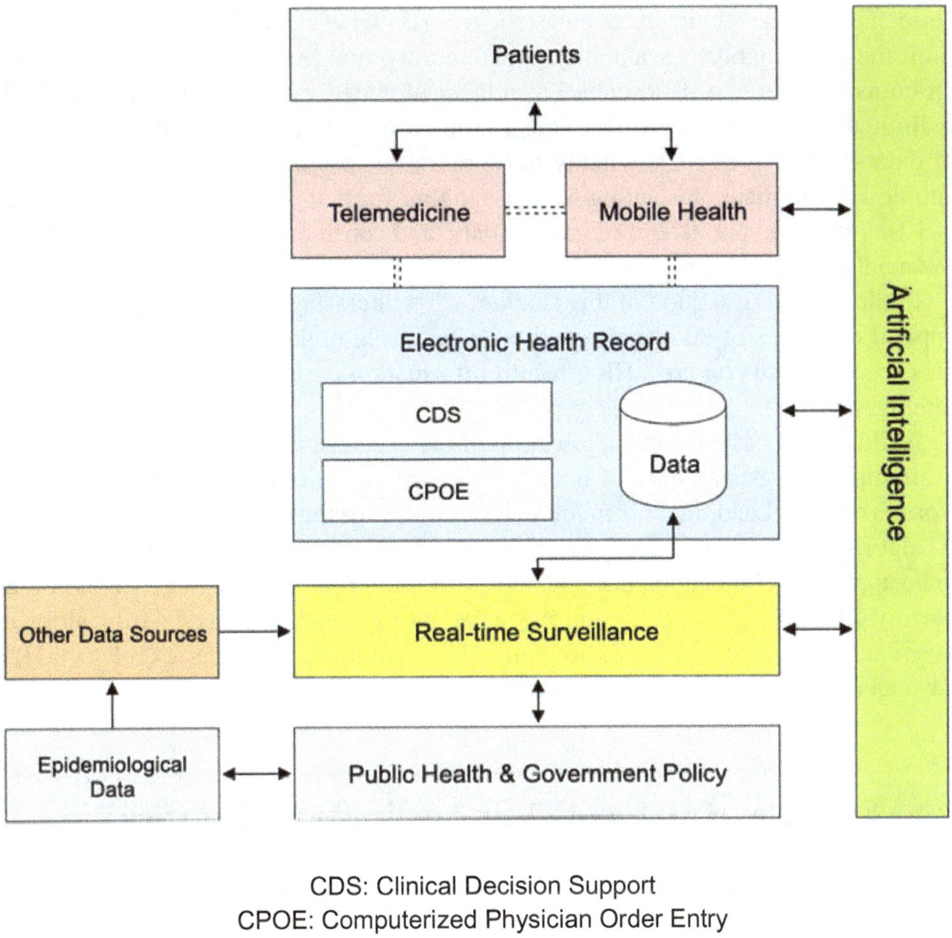

Fig. 1.1 Elements of healthcare information technology

stakeholders in the care process—from the healthcare leaders and managers over healthcare professionals to patients and communities (Al-Shorbaji 2018).

However, uptake of these technologies has been uneven within and across countries due to differing levels of maturity in ICT infrastructure, lack of skilled healthcare personnel, and more. These are often among the fundamental hurdles in updating and maintaining up-to-date HIT, especially in low and middle-income countries (LMICs) (Clifford 2016). In several countries, however, various pilot implementations have been initiated but few have gone to scale (Sundin et al. 2016). This was due to several factors with socio-cultural challenges at the core despite great financial, clinical, and logistical enablement from supporting organizations and responsible governments (Clifford 2016). Additionally, countries, particularly LMICs, continue to be challenged by the rapid development of HIT interventions, such as constantly evolving EHR infrastructures. Successful adoption and implementation of HIT solutions are also constrained by other challenges such as poor ICT infrastructure and access, misalignment between HIT investments and the national health agenda, and poorly defined enterprise architectures and standards (Baller et al. 2016). All of these factors limit the accountability, scalability, sustainability, and resilience of health systems. Of course, the role of data science as a layer of added value, enabled through HIT, is limited in settings where HIT integration is low. On the other hand, the impact of data science in LMICs is likely to be more far-reaching with the integration of simple HIT applications, acting as low-hanging fruits to improve care (Costa et al. 2012). Yet it is imperative to remain realistic and consider the structural, social, and financial obstacles we are faced with.

In the following section of this chapter, we will closely examine three frequently applied examples of HIT and how these play a role in data science. The technologies we will focus on are EHRs, health information exchange (HIE), and artificial intelligence (AI).

Building the basis for the application of data science techniques by enabling the availability of vasts amount of data, EHRs display a means for the collection and storage of data. Leading on from here, HIE allows for the exchange of this data, and AI algorithms will subsequently grant the analysis and provision of predictive models to be applied in clinical practice and administration. Hence, these three technologies portray different aspects of the journey a patient's clinical data takes—from storage, over exchange, to analysis. Additionally, they symbolize examples of relevant HIT advancements over the years in a chronological manner.

1.2 Examples of HIT and Their Application in Data Science

1.2.1 Applied Example No. 1: Electronic Health Records (EHRs)

One of the key prerequisites for improving the delivery of care services through data science is the efficient collection, storage, analysis, and exchange of health information across different service levels in a secure yet practical fashion. Data science tools, such as machine learning and deep learning, rely heavily on massive collections of labelled structured and unstructured data, in order to train models and subsequently improve them to guide decision. Hence, a data acquisition pipeline is paramount. For this purpose, EHRs have become indispensable tools to carry patient health information and facilitate its use between different levels of care. This is reflected by the increasing number of national HIT strategies around the globe, starring the implementation and development of EHR systems (World Health Organization 2016).

High income countries have seen the largest investments in EHR systems. In the United States, the Health Information Technology for Economic and Clinical Health Act (HITECH Act of 2009) spurred on the rapid digitization of the healthcare delivery system, eventually culminating in the Medicare and Medicaid EHR Incentive Programs (Washington et al. 2017). Here, EHRs have provided accurate and up-to-date information at the point of care, enabled quicker access to patient records for more coordinated care among healthcare providers, and reduced healthcare costs by decreasing the amount of paperwork and duplicate diagnostic exams while streamlining coding and billing services as a result of complete and accurate documentation of all transactions.

However, the adoption and implementation of EHRs have been a great source of both satisfaction and consternation, particularly in the last ten years. In recent years, physicians' satisfaction with EHRs have become universally low (Shanafelt et al. 2016), probably due to an increasing workload and the incentives received as a result of complete documentation. Unintentionally, this has gradually become a burden for providers around the world by negatively affecting their relationship with patients and clinical workflows (Goldberg 2018). In 2016, a study by Shanafelt, et al., revealed that physicians who used EHRs and computerized physician order entry (CPOE) systems, *e.g.*, electronic prescribing, demonstrated a lower level of work satisfaction due to the amount of time spent on clerical tasks and had an increased risk of burnout (Shanafelt et al. 2016). Moreover, physicians have progressively become concerned that medical malpractice liability may increase with the implementation of CPOE systems due to the increased documentation of computer-related errors (Mangalmurti et al. 2010). In LMICs, this set of problems could prove even more troublesome as the working conditions for health professionals are likely to be even more challenging. Adding an EHR system without taking into consideration all its implications could have disastrous consequences for all aspects of care provision and staff satisfaction.

Further examples of this ambivalence are tools that count as subordinate functions of EHRs, including CPOE systems and Clinical Decision Support (CDS) systems. As mentioned above, electronic prescribing is one prominent example of a CPOE system. As opposed to handwritten prescriptions, the electronic prescribing alternative promises greater prevention of medication errors. Reasons for this are increased completeness, standardization, and legibility of pharmaceutical prescriptions, as well as their frequent integration with CDS tools (Puaar and Franklin 2017). CDS systems are digital applications to "provide alerts, reminders, prescribing recommendations, therapeutic guidelines, image interpretation, and diagnostic assistance" (Khairat et al. 2018) and are often deployed to complement CPOE systems. This integration leads to an enhancement of patient safety with lower prescriptions errors and improved interprofessional communication between healthcare providers (Mills et al. 2017).

However, despite the proven potential of CDS for electronic drug alerts by reducing the number of adverse drug events and lowering healthcare costs (Ash et al. 2007); (Weingart et al. 2009), it is one of the leading causes of alert fatigue in healthcare providers. Alert fatigue describes a phenomenon where the user, *i.e.* the clinician, actively ignores or dismisses pop-up windows, warning the user of possible errors or dangers with clinical information that they entered. Alerts for drug-drug interactions, pre-existing drug allergies, weight-adjusted dosing etc., often appear very frequently, hence 'fatiguing' the user's attention to them (Backman et al. 2017). It has been shown to debilitate the power of alerts, especially if deemed obvious or irrelevant, leading clinicians to dismiss future pop-ups without reading potentially important alert messages (Ash et al. 2007). Consequences of alert fatigue could lead to the user's impression of being supervised and treated as distrusted in their own decision-making with resentment due to the continuous interruption in their work. In order to prevent this, it is therefore imperative to ensure user-friendliness, along with the relevance and appropriateness of alerts in the given clinical context when designing CDS systems (Ash et al. 2007).

Considering these benefits and drawbacks of EHRs, along with CPOE and CDS, that are inherent to their integration, they certainly all allow for the further collection of data by the digitization and integration of workflows, such as the prescription of medication. Before the integration of HIT, these processes either used to be analogue or non-existent, whereas now they can be streamlined and interoperable with one another. This may ease the documentation burden of handwritten notes and enable the collection of even more clinical data, which can much more readily find application for research or in public health. However, as with all technological novelties in healthcare, if not integrated well, all systems can become cumbersome and in several ways harmful to deliver good care. Healthcare professionals may circumvent the correct use of these electronic systems, which may negatively impact overall efficiency, effectiveness of care, and patient safety (Blijleven et al. 2017).

The full impact of EHRs on data science in global health is challenged by smaller and larger scale problems, ranging from human issues to technical difficulties. It begins with the above mentioned issues, *e.g.*, low EHR usability and staff resistance, and ends with the major, systems-based problems of healthcare, such as the increase in healthcare cost, the rate of medical errors, or exhaustion and shortage of workforce, all of which limit the integration and adequate maintenance of EHR systems.

1.2.2 Applied Example No. 2: Health Information Exchange (HIE)

Health information exchange (HIE) is the mobilization and transfer of electronic health information within and across organizations in a community, region, or country, ideally through interoperable health information systems (Finn 2011). It allows healthcare providers and patients to securely access medical information electronically in order to appropriately and confidentially share patient's health information independent of where they are receiving care (HealthIT.gov 2017). The United States, Canada, Australia, and the UK are some of the countries who have, to a certain extent, successfully implemented regional or state-wide HIEs.

An effective implementation of HIE is critical to provide high-quality, tailored care to patients while reducing costs and increasing access (Sadoughi et al. 2018). To do this, HIE implementation must be aligned with inner-organizational as well as inter-organizational needs and priorities, with mutual cooperation and collaboration being crucial in fostering HIE. In 2016, Eden, et al., showed that facilitators and barriers to successful HIE implementation could be categorized as to the completeness of information, organization and workflow, and technology and user needs (Eden et al.

2016). In particular, the lack of consistent terminology and classification of HIE was found to be a considerable barrier to understanding how an HIE ideally functions, as well as constant changes in sociotechnical systems (Eden et al. 2016). These findings are consistent with the 2016 study of Akhlaq, et al., done for LMICs, wherein they found that successful HIE implementations largely depend on effective policies, strong leadership, and governance in order to create an evidence-based decision-making culture within organizations (Akhlaq et al. 2016).

Revisiting the concept of EHRs and thinking a step ahead, being able to not only access local clinical data but to exchange data across departments, organizations, regions, or even nations through HIEs, a whole new extent of data availability becomes apparent. Due to these vast amounts of data being necessary in order to leverage its full potential, it symbolizes a key requirement for data science adding real-world value and effectively integrate AI on a broader scale. Still being far from achieving a smooth and widespread HIE across regions and countries, for the most part, we can only speculate on the impact the analysis of all this data can have once this will be achieved. As a result of these HIE networks, we need to find the value of all the accumulated data, not only by making medical practice more evidence-based but also in the field of, *e.g.*, population-based informatics, or genetic and genomic information. Generally, once data is available, analysing it and drawing conclusions from it for clinical practice is relatively easy as compared to the far greater hurdle of translating these findings from 'bench to bedside'.

Taking another step ahead, blockchain technology (*for more details, please refer to subsequent chapters of this book*) has been proposed as a tool to provide the necessary features for long sought after advancements in the industry, especially with regard to increased interoperability, high data security, and seamless HIE (Gordon and Catalini 2018). Similarly, a good amount of temperance may also be needed. Blockchain has been envisioned to change the status quo in clinical research, public health, patient identification systems, and self-generated health data (Gordon et al. 2017). It has also been explored in terms of improving global health (Metcalf 2019, p. 415). However, one has to keep in mind that health systems are multifaceted, highly fragmented, and very resistant to change. Thus, expectations should be kept realistic in the face of persistent doubts on its sectoral need, appropriate use, and whether it can truly change existing health systems—particularly on data handling, because of the lack of scalable real-world implementations (Gordon et al. 2017).

Besides the necessary technological prerequisites, key to the successful implementation of an HIE are governance, consistency in technical nomenclature, and effective change management. These three factors are determined to have significant effects on the level of adoption and success that organizations experience when implementing an HIE. As they are extremely difficult to achieve due to the need for many disparate parties to align, conferences can foster the conversations that enable broader and effective change management, bringing all different stakeholders to the table. It outlines the need for collaboration as health data, if collected in an orderly and accessible fashion, is still mostly siloed unless governance and other initiatives drive parties towards unification and liberation of data.

1.2.3 Applied Example No. 3: Artificial Intelligence

Given that EHRs and HIE have done their work to provide data in an accessible and orderly fashion so that it can be further utilized, artificial intelligence (AI) can be applied in helping to improve everyday clinical questions, predict disease outbreaks in LMICs, monitor drug adherence, etc. The application of these new technologies have spurred excitement and brought renewed hope in finding solutions to the intricate and sophisticated problems inherent to global health.

With AI applied to healthcare and global health, we associate the use of computer algorithms and statistical models to enhance the human understanding of complicated medical information and coherences by analyzing medical data. Specifically, AI usually refers to tasks performed by computers that would otherwise require intelligence if executed by humans (The Alan Turing Institute 2018).

The field of AI has evolved over the last 60 years. First described in 1971 in medical publications (Coiera 1996), it is only now that many AI applications have been deployed in healthcare settings and there are signs indicating that AI adoption has been growing exponentially. Areas that would benefit from added value through data-driven solutions can be classified as having either a 'patient focus' and/or 'healthcare provider/payers focus' (Garbuio and Lin 2019). Within clinical medicine, as part of the latter focus, there is a myriad of specialties that would benefit from the integration of AI engines, with possible tasks ranging from natural language processing over clinical decision support to predictive analytics (Dankwa-Mullan et al. 2018); (Yu and Kohane 2018) (*for more details, please refer to subsequent chapters of this book*). Despite the fact that a range of those AI applications have already proven to perform on par with experienced clinical specialists (Esteva et al. 2017), many experts see AI's future role in complementing human knowledge and decisions, by rapidly exploiting vasts amount of data, instead of replacing doctors (Dankwa-Mullan et al. 2018). Hence, most AI applications in healthcare are aimed at working in synergy with staff instead of striving for a substitution of workforce.

One major application of AI-assisted medicine is the ability to make reliable and accurate predictions on clinical outcomes, hence assisting clinicians in critical everyday decisions, for example by finding the optimal treatment strategy for patients with sepsis (Komorowski et al. 2018) or utilizing warning algorithms and severity of illness scores in intensive care (AIMed 2018). Other examples include radiological or pathological image processing through deep neural networks (Esteva et al. 2017). Hence, machine learning and deep learning, methods of AI, will not only alleviate a great portion of physicians' workload but will also provide more accurate clinical prognoses and enhance diagnostic accuracy (Obermeyer and Emanuel 2016). This triad of features ultimately contributes to ML enhancing patients' outcomes with the adoption of AI in healthcare.

An industry example of an AI application currently in use for global health is IDx, a US-based startup. The company has succeeded in building the first and only FDA authorized AI system for the autonomous detection of retinopathy in adults with diabetes, namely IDx-DR (FDA, 2018). The shift towards AI oriented efforts is also being demonstrated by academia, *e.g.*, with the foundation of the Stanford Institute for Human-Centered Artificial Intelligence in early 2019. Other academic examples include free online courses, like MIT's course "Global Health Informatics to Improve Quality of Care" on edX (Celi 2019) or Stanford's Andrew Ng's course in Machine Learning on Coursera, enabling anyone to gain an understanding of health informatics and how to leverage Big Data (Ng 2011).

However, despite all the excitement and the predicted opportunities for bettering healthcare using AI, bringing ML algorithms from a laboratory to the bedside remains a major challenge. Regulatory and ethical issues, such as confirmatory bias or reduced patient safety, have been discussed involving the routine use of AI, with uncertainty regarding the point of sufficient performance of a program and accountability in the event of a medical error (Dankwa-Mullan et al., 2018). The absence of such controlling mechanisms to date raises questions as to whether the use of AI, though it may solve problems and enhance care delivery, may again create new unintended problems, such as reducing efficiency (Yu and Kohane 2018) or questionable clinical success rates of new algorithms, leading to concerns for patient safety.

1.3 Discussion

With all of the challenges faced by current global healthcare systems, including an ever-increasing financial burden and an aging population, the use of HIT systems and data science have the potential to improve the effectiveness of treatments while reducing costs and increasing the quality of care, as suggested by many studies (Silow-Carroll et al. 2012); (Murphy 2014); (Sadoughi et al. 2018). Moreover, they may not only enable a more holistic patient care by facilitating collaboration among different service providers but have the potential to improve patients' and providers' experience and satisfaction. Aside from alleviating patients' own burden in receiving appropriate care, the clinicians' experience may also likely be enhanced when care becomes again more efficacious and patient-focused, *e.g.*, when medical records are easily accessible, prescriptions errors would be flagged before having negative effects, or algorithms could give specific treatment recommendations in the management of complex clinical conditions. In an ideal situation, appropriately applied HIT can reduce clinicians' workload and reverse the increased documentation burden to make physicians' work more patient-centered again with more time allowed for face-to-face interaction, increasing both patient and staff satisfaction. This is more the case in LMICs where these modalities could offer the opportunity to leapfrog in achieving Universal Health Coverage.

Despite all the benefits and advantages that these technologies deliver, one must also consider potential problems that halt, or arise from, their integration: Healthcare systems are extremely rigid to change, many stakeholders have very disparate or misaligned incentives, there is resilience towards change and reluctance by users, there is a global increase in the demand of care leading to rising costs, all of which is paired with persisting difficulties of data fragmentation and lacking HIT interoperability. These factors display significant barriers that must be overcome in order to drive change in the right direction. As the challenges are multifactorial, multi-faceted teams are required to tackle them. This requires a culture change to overhaul long-established operational processes and workflows, which are highly complex and involve a host of actors, in order to work towards optimal digitalization. Newly arising problems, such as interoperability issues between varied health information systems established in isolation, continue to be a substantial challenge for a smooth information exchange. On top of this, the integration of new technologies to solve old problems paves the way for new problems to arise. These revolve not only around financial implications (*e.g.*, maintenance costs) but also around regulatory and ethical issues. As with IDx-DR, the U.S. Department of Health and Human Services for Food and Drug Administration (FDA) has approved their algorithm as medical device and granted its unsupervised use (Van Der Heijden et al. 2018). However, AI algorithms function differently to what was traditionally defined as medical device, because they must constantly evolve to maintain their accuracy. This high amount of uncertainty demands great attention for a regulatory and ethical debate going forward. In the global context, this might give rise to an increase in health disparity between the have and the have-not.

The complexity of challenges that health systems are faced with increases. Despite data science bringing hope to solve many long-established problems in the face of aforementioned difficulties in the smooth collection, exchange, and subsequent analysis of data, bringing change from bench to bedside cannot be done by technology alone and involves mainly human factors. The rise of algorithms to enhance medical diagnosis and decision-making are only of value when they are being implemented in day-to-day practice and accessible to the entire global community. In this regard, the efforts of organizations, such as Sana (MIT), are of paramount importance in promoting data science in global health (Angelidis et al. 2016).

1.4 Conclusion

In order to universally improve healthcare, countries need to balance cost, quality, and access, and HIT has proven to have the potential in addressing these needs. Using it and applying principles of data science allows information to be stored, processed, exchanged, and analyzed in order to maximize its value and use. If used effectively, it can lead to a more efficient and safe delivery of care, improved access to information and services for an evidence-based decision-making, and enhance both clinicians' and patients' satisfaction. However, the necessary HIT requires a conducive ICT-enabled environment in order to facilitate the greatest possible degree of interoperability and cross-disciplinary collaboration.

All technological advancements and their possibilities are of limited use, however, when they cannot be implemented and utilized effectively due to a misalignment with the human layer. For example, when designing HIT applications, the user experience must be equally important as its anticipated improvement in clinical effectiveness and efficiency. Likewise must stakeholders communicate through agreed terminology and work towards a common goal. This can only be achieved by an evenly close collaboration of software developers with future users, governments with healthcare managers, and data scientists with clinicians. Especially in the context of LMICs, joint forces between professions and regions are likely to have better outcomes than many individual efforts to innovate healthcare. Here, governmental drive can be an important initiating force in fostering the necessary interprofessional partnerships, which should ideally go beyond organizational or regional interests.

The utilization of data science has the potential to tackle some of the greatest challenges in modern healthcare that exist on various different levels, eventually contributing to making advancements in global health. Although, in order for HIT applications to function as they have been designed currently and will be designed in the future, all stakeholders need to collaborate in tackling technical, behavioural, financial, ethical, and regulatory challenges to enable the best possible use of these technologies for leveraging data science in global health.

References

AIMed, B. (2018). The ethical imperative of learning from the data—AI Med [WWW document]. AI Med. Retrieved October 22, 2018, from http://ai-med.io/the-ethical-imperative-of-learning-from-the-data/.

Akhlaq, A., McKinstry, B., Muhammad, K. B., & Sheikh, A. (2016). Barriers and facilitators to health information exchange in low- and middle-income country settings: A systematic review. *Health Policy and Planning, 31,* 1310–1325.

Al-Shorbaji, N. (2018). The world health assembly resolutions on eHealth: eHealth in support of universal health coverage. *Methods of Information in Medicine, 52,* 463–466.

Angelidis, P., Berman, L., Casas-Perez, M. de la, L., Celi, L. A., Dafoulas, G. E., Dagan, A., Escobar, B., Lopez, D. M., Noguez, J., Osorio-Valencia, J. S., Otine, C., Paik, K., Rojas-Potosi, L., Symeonidis, A. L., Winkler, E. (2016). The hackathon model to spur innovation around global mHealth. *Journal of Medical Engineering & Technology, 40,* 392–399.

Ash, J. S., Sittig, D. F., Campbell, E. M., Guappone, K. P., Dykstra, R. H. (2007). Some unintended consequences of clinical decision support systems. *AMIA Annual Symposium Proceedings,* 26–30.

Backman, R., Bayliss, S., Moore, D., & Litchfield, I. (2017). Clinical reminder alert fatigue in healthcare: A systematic literature review protocol using qualitative evidence. *Systematic Review, 6,* 255.

Baller, S., Dutta, S., & Lanvin, B. (2016). *The global information technology report 2016.* World Economic Forum.

Blijleven, V., Koelemeijer, K., Wetzels, M., & Jaspers, M. (2017). Workarounds emerging from electronic health record system usage: Consequences for patient safety, effectiveness of care, and efficiency of care. *JMIR Hum Factors, 4,* e27.

Celi, L. A. (2019). Global health informatics to improve quality of care [WWW document]. edX. Retrieved April 17, 2019 https://www.edx.org/course/global-health-informatics-to-improve-quality-of-care.

Clifford, G. D. (2016). E-health in low to middle income countries. *Journal of Medical Engineering & Technology, 40,* 336–341.

Coiera, E. W. (1996). Artificial intelligence in medicine: The challenges ahead. *Journal of the American Medical Informatics Association, 3,* 363–366.

Costa, C. M., Gondim, D. D., Gondim, D. D., Soares, H. B., Ribeiro, A. G. C. D., Silva, I., et al. (2012). S2DIA: A diagnostic system for diabetes mellitus using SANA platform. *Conference on Proceedings of IEEE Engineering in Medicine and Biology Society, 2012,* 6078–6081.

Dankwa-Mullan, I., Rivo, M., Sepulveda, M., Park, Y., Snowdon, J., & Rhee, K. (2018). Transforming diabetes care through artificial intelligence: The future is here. *Population Health Management.*

Eden, K. B., Totten, A. M., Kassakian, S. Z., Gorman, P. N., McDonagh, M. S., Devine, B., et al. (2016). Barriers and facilitators to exchanging health information: A systematic review. *International Journal of Medical Informatics, 88,* 44–51.

Esteva, A., Kuprel, B., Novoa, R. A., Ko, J., Swetter, S. M., Blau, H. M., et al. (2017). Dermatologist-level classification of skin cancer with deep neural networks. *Nature, 542,* 115–118.

FDA. (2018). FDA news release—FDA permits marketing of artificial intelligence-based device to detect certain diabetes-related eye problems [WWW document]. U.S. Food and Drug Administration. Retrieved April 4, 2019, from https://www.fda.gov/newsevents/newsroom/pressannouncements/ucm604357.htm.

Finn, N. (2011). *Health information exchange: a stepping stone toward continuity of care and participatory medicine.* Med: J. Particip.

Garbuio, M., & Lin, N. (2019). Artificial intelligence as a growth engine for health care startups: Emerging business models. *California Management Review, 61,* 59–83.

Goldberg, D. J. (2018). The burden of electronic health record implementation [WWW document]. *Dermatology Times.* Retrieved November 11, 2018, from http://www.dermatologytimes.com/legal-eagle/will-dr-emr-have-more-or-less-liability-his-new-electronic-health-records.

Gordon, W. J., Catalini, C. (2018). Blockchain technology for healthcare: Facilitating the transition to patient-driven interoperability [WWW document]. Retrieved October 22, 2018, from https://www.ncbi.nlm.nih.gov/pubmed/30069284.

Gordon, W., Wright, A., Landman, A. (2017). Blockchain in health care: Decoding the hype [WWW document]. NEJM catalyst. Retrieved October 22, 2018, from https://catalyst.nejm.org/decoding-blockchain-technology-health/.

HealthIT.gov. (2017). Health information exchange [WWW document]. HealthIT.gov—Health IT and health information exchange basics: health information exchange. Retrieved November 18, 2018, from https://www.healthit.gov/topic/health-it-basics/health-information-exchange.

Khairat, S., Marc, D., Crosby, W., & Al Sanousi, A. (2018). Reasons For Physicians Not Adopting Clinical Decision Support Systems: Critical Analysis. *JMIR Med Inform, 6,* e24.

Komorowski, M., Celi, L. A., Badawi, O., Gordon, A. C., & Faisal, A. A. (2018). The artificial intelligence clinician learns optimal treatment strategies for sepsis in intensive care. *Nature Medicine, 24,* 1716–1720.

Koplan, J. P., Bond, T. C., Merson, M. H., Reddy, K. S., Rodriguez, M. H., Sewankambo, N. K., Wasserheit, J. N. (2009). Consortium of universities for global health executive board. Towards a common definition of global health. *Lancet, 373,* 1993–1995.

Mangalmurti, S. S., Murtagh, L., & Mello, M. M. (2010). Medical malpractice liability in the age of electronic health records. *New England Journal of Medicine, 363,* 2060–2067.

Metcalf, D. (2019). *Blockchain in healthcare: Innovations that empower patients, connect professionals and improve care.* Taylor & Francis.

Mills, P. R., Weidmann, A. E., & Stewart, D. (2017). Hospital staff views of prescribing and discharge communication before and after electronic prescribing system implementation. *International Journal of Clinical Pharmacy, 39,* 1320–1330.

Murphy, E. V. (2014). Clinical decision support: Effectiveness in improving quality processes and clinical outcomes and factors that may influence success. *Yale Journal of Biology and Medicine, 87,* 187–197.

Ng, A. (2011). Machine learning [WWW Document]. Coursera. Retrieved 17 April, 2019, from https://www.coursera.org/learn/machine-learning.

Obermeyer, Z., & Emanuel, E. J. (2016). Predicting the future—Big data, machine learning, and clinical medicine. *New England Journal of Medicine, 375,* 1216–1219.

Puaar, S. J., & Franklin, B. D. (2017). Impact of an inpatient electronic prescribing system on prescribing error causation: A qualitative evaluation in an English hospital. *BMJ Quality Safety, 27,* 529–538.

Sadoughi, F., Nasiri, S., & Ahmadi, H. (2018). The impact of health information exchange on healthcare quality and cost-effectiveness: A systematic literature review. *Computer Methods and Programs in Biomedicine, 161,* 209–232.

Shanafelt, T. D., Dyrbye, L. N., Sinsky, C., Hasan, O., Satele, D., Sloan, J., et al. (2016). Relationship between clerical burden and characteristics of the electronic environment with physician burnout and professional satisfaction. *Mayo Clinic Proceedings, 91,* 836–848.

Silow-Carroll, S., Edwards, J. N., & Rodin, D. (2012). Using electronic health records to improve quality and efficiency: The experiences of leading hospitals. *Issue Brief, 17,* 1–40.

Singh, H., & Sittig, D. F. (2016). Measuring and improving patient safety through health information technology: The health IT safety framework. *BMJ Quality & Safety, 25,* 226–232.

Sundin, P., Callan, J., & Mehta, K. (2016). Why do entrepreneurial mHealth ventures in the developing world fail to scale? *Journal of Medical Engineering & Technology, 40,* 444–457.

The Alan Turing Institute. (2018). The Alan turing institute. Retrieved October 22, 2018, from https://www.turing.ac.uk.

Van Der Heijden, A. A., Abramoff, M. D., Verbraak, F., van Hecke, M. V., Liem, A., & Nijpels, G. (2018). Validation of automated screening for referable diabetic retinopathy with the IDx-DR device in the Hoorn diabetes care system. *Acta Ophthalmologica, 96,* 63–68.

Washington, V., DeSalvo, K., Mostashari, F., & Blumenthal, D. (2017). The HITECH era and the path forward. *New England Journal of Medicine, 377,* 904–906.

Weingart, S. N., Simchowitz, B., Padolsky, H., Isaac, T., Seger, A. C., Massagli, M., et al. (2009). An empirical model to estimate the potential impact of medication safety alerts on patient safety, health care utilization, and cost in ambulatory care. *Archives of Internal Medicine, 169,* 1465–1473.

World Health Assembly. (2005). WHA58.28 eHealth.

World Health Organization. (2013). *The world health report 2013: Research for universal health coverage.* World Health Organization.

World Health Organization. (2016). *Atlas of eHealth country profiles 2015: The use of eHealth in support of universal health coverage Based on the findings of the 2015 global survey on eHealth.* World Health Organization.

Yu, K.-H., Kohane, I. S. (2018). Framing the challenges of artificial intelligence in medicine. *BMJ Quality & Safety bmjqs* 2018–008551.

2

Role of Design Thinking in Solving Challenges Related to Frail Elderly People

Tony Gallanis

Abstract Design thinking is a valuable, iterative process to utilize when building an innovation. Rather than starting from a singular novel technology in search of a problem, the design thinking approach begins with assessing the environment, users, and stakeholders, attempting to identify alternative strategies and solutions. This process generally leads to a more holistic and sustainable intervention, improving outcomes and adoption. This chapter provides a primer to design thinking, as well an introductory toolkit to begin applying the approach to your innovations.

Keywords Design thinking · Innovation · Desirability · Feasibility · Empathy · Ideation

Learning Objectives: In this chapter, we will explore the process of design thinking as a discipline. We will then explore its integration within healthcare. By the end of the chapter, a reader shall be able to:

- Define the concept of design thinking
- Examine the intersection between design thinking and innovation
- Identify the role of empathy in the design thinking process
- List the tools that are useful to embed design thinking in global health projects
- Apply design thinking to tackle a global health challenge.

2.1 Design Thinking Introduction

Innovations are seen to be bold, new, creative solutions to problems. Often, these innovative solutions require an explicit understanding of the problem that needs to be solved from the user's perspective. This approach to drive innovation—coined Design Thinking—requires discipline and is often different than the way most people conduct traditional problem-solving. Traditionally, innovation projects result from a team gathering together, creating specifications for the innovation, and fulfilling

T. Gallanis (✉)
MIT Critical Data, 77 Massachusetts, Avenue E25-505, Cambridge, MA 02139, USA
e-mail: gallanistg@gmail.com

the specifications within the allocated budget. Design thinking differs by allowing the specifications to be driven by the user's needs and the nature of the problem. Design thinking has been the linchpin of the tech and startup ecosystem in the recent decade. Still, the problem-first nature of design thinking is applicable beyond the startup world and has the potential to provide the global health workforce with better tools to work through the most challenging of global health dilemmas. Design thinking digs quickly to the root cause of a problem and provides tools and resources for teams to then create powerful solutions. In the following chapter, we will address how design thinking can match the unmet need for user-driven innovation in global health and how global health practitioners can embed this disciplined approach to support global health initiatives.

2.1.1 Design Thinking Workshop for Global Health

Addressing air pollution, noncommunicable diseases, potential influenza pandemics, high threat pathogens, ageing society, and weak healthcare systems are among some of the several profound challenges in global health (WHO 2019a). Aging societies pose numerous challenges to global health. Around the world, populations are aging at a faster rate than before. By 2050, the over 60 age demographic will more than double, reaching 2 billion people. With the rising population of older adults, geriatric syndromes will increase in prevalence causing strain on the healthcare system to treat more dementia, hearing loss, cataracts, back and neck pain, and diabetes (WHO 2018). Already, dementia among older adults is an $800 billion challenge that causes strain on healthcare systems, caregivers, and those affected by the illness (WHO 2019b). Aging societies need bold solutions to address the health needs of older adults. Each of these challenges is daunting due to the complexity of the problem and scope of the intervention required to effect positive change. Challenges that are vast and imposing are often those best poised to benefit from design thinking. This chapter is based on the lessons learned using design thinking during a Global Health Datathon organized at the Khon Kaen University in Thailand. The Datathon worked through one of the many challenges in global health—aging societies—and applied design thinking to bring about solutions for three different users who vary in frailty severity.

For participants of the Khon Kaen University (KKU) Datathon workshop that inspired this chapter, the design focus was on understanding problems faced by frail older adults. Frailty refers to the clinically recognizable state of an older adult who is vulnerable for severe complications or injuries. The frailty phenotype, as put forth by Fried et al., is commonly denoted as a combination of three of the five following traits: physical weakness, slow walking, low physical activity, low energy, or weight loss (WHO 2016). The challenges experienced by frail adults are many since frail population are at elevated risk for falls, hospitalizations, and mortality (Ensrud et al. 2007).

2.1.2 Overview of the Workshop

The workshop was composed of two sessions. During the first, participants learned vital tools and methods of design thinking. Design methods are frameworks and tools used to shape one's workflow and mindset through the course of the design thinking process (Jones 1992). The second session focused on the application of those tools within the context of the challenge of ageing. The total length of the KKU Datathon workshop was 3 hours with a short break in the middle. Participants ranged in age from university students to older executives. The backgrounds of participants included data scientists, clinicians, researchers, public health workers, nurses, and administrators. There were approximately 25 participants in attendance. A PowerPoint presentation was used to guide participants through the design thinking workshop. Markers, easel-pads, and sticky notes were provided for participants to work through the applied portion of the workshop. Like the workshop, this chapter first will focus on design methods and then apply them to the design challenge: the experience of frail, older adults.

2.2 Part I: Introduction to Design Thinking

2.2.1 General Overview

Design thinking is a process with mindsets to navigate uncertainty and arrive at insightful innovations (IDEO 2019). Design thinking mindsets are ways for the designer, as the practitioner of design thinking, to approach the problem and the various stages of design thinking. Mindsets guide the designer on how to embrace the problem and where to look for inspirations and solutions.

Often, people assume design thinking to be the holy grail of innovation. Simply employ design thinking and innovations will spontaneously spring forth, but this is not the case (Nussbaum 2011). As a disciple of design thinking, it is important to first to indulge the mindsets that unleash one's creative confidence and second to ensure the space and support to employ innovative work through design thinking. Simply following the design thinking process will not bring about the intended innovations. One must buy into the processes with certain thoughtfulness to build one's creative confidence (Kelley et al. 2019). Secondly, support systems, buy-in from leadership, diversity of skillsets, space for working, and time to create are all key ingredients in fostering the right ecosystem for design thinking (Waters 2011).

2.2.2 *Defining Innovation*

Innovation in design thinking is the intersection of desirability, feasibility, and viability. Desirability refers to the user's want for the product or offering at hand. Feasibility refers to the ability of the team to create the product. Viability refers to the sustainability of the solution. The intersection of desirability, feasibility, and viability is innovation (IDEO 2019) (Fig. 2.1).

One caveat in the definition of innovation employed by designers is the expressed prioritization of desirability over feasibility and viability. In global health, one could constrain the innovation to whether it was feasible given the resources on hand or whether it would be viable after implementation. When designers prioritize desirability chiefly among the three, designers are hinting that it may be more beneficial to build an innovation that addresses a person's needs rather than an innovation that can be allocated funding or be built with available resources. One of the fatal flaws of innovation teams is the creation of things that do not serve real problems. This fatal flaw has vast repercussions in global health. Occasionally, governing bodies, non-profit organizations, or ministries of health may be keen on implementing a solution, but the solution itself may not address a real need for the intended user. This problem leads to a solution that is not desired by the target population.

During the West African Ebola outbreak in 2014 as well as the recent 2019 Congo Ebola outbreak, occasionally all-white personal protective equipment (PPE) was used by frontline health workers when treating Ebola patients. All-white PPE conjured notions of ghosts and death, notions that hindered the ability of frontline health workers to treat patients (UNICEF 2019). Frontline health workers who donned the

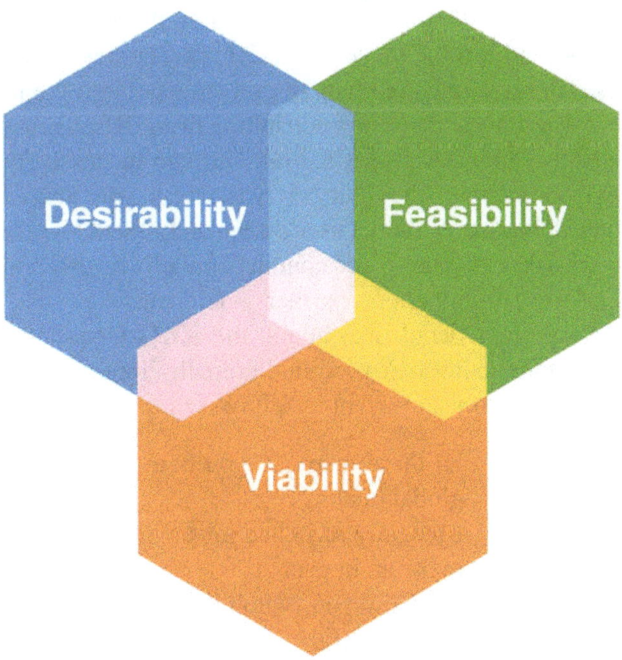

Fig. 2.1 Innovation intersection

all-white PPE would instill fear in their patients during treatment. Patients would fear the frontline health workers who traveled into towns to extract sickly patients or avoid treatment altogether. In this scenario, the actions of the frontline health workers were hindered because patients did not desire the treatment provided. The nature of the Ebola epidemic was perceived to be one of patients not receiving medical care when the true nature of the problem was patients not finding comfort and security in the treatment available. A proposed solution to the challenge of comfort and security of the patient during the treatment process was the PPE Portrait Project. The PPE Portrait Project taped a portrait of the frontline health worker's face to the outside of the all-white PPE. With the portrait adorned on the front of the PPE, patients could see the humanity of the person behind the ghostly white suit. This humanity connected the patient and the frontline health worker to lessen fears of treatment. The PPE Portrait Project taped a portrait of the worker to the outside of the PPE, enabling patients to connect with the frontline health workers and alleviate fears (Heffernan 2019; Crossan 2015).

2.2.3 Developing Empathy

Empathy is critical in the design thinking process, especially when a designer places an explicit emphasis on the desirability of an innovation. In design thinking, empathy is the process of uncovering the desires and aspirations of the users for the intended product or service. Without researching and learning what a user truly struggles accomplishing, a designer will be unable to know how to create a desirable innovation.

There are many ways to conduct empathy research and the methods parallel other qualitative research methods including those of ethnographic research and primary market research (Reeves et al. 2008). The key to empathy research is to engage a user in some way and then to probe deeper into the user's perspective. One strategy employed by a top design consulting firm, IDEO, is to conduct The Five Whys during an interview (Design Kit 2019a). Through successively asking the user why they acted in a certain way, the interviewer is able to peel away at the internal motivations and underpinnings behind a user's actions. In the KKU Datathon workshop, participants were asked to pair up and conduct empathy research in the form of 1 on 1 interviews. For three minutes one partner would interview the other person to uncover why their partner decided to attend the KKU Datathon workshop on design thinking and global health. A profound empathy interview that occurred during a different Datathon workshop went as follows:

Participant Hi there, **why** are you here at this workshop on design thinking and global health?

Interviewee I recently switched jobs from finance to healthcare and am hoping to make an impact.

Participant **Why** did you switch jobs to healthcare?

Interviewee My previous job became dull over time and I felt disconnected to people.

Participant **Why** do you desire to be connected to people?

Interviewee There's something special about getting to know people's health challenges and finding ways to help.

Participant **Why** is it so special?

Interviewee It's not every day that someone opens up to you about their struggles, so you have to make the most of it when they do.

Participant **Why** do you have to make the most of it?

Interviewee Well, someone helped me through a hard time and, I guess, I just want to do the same.

Without conducting an empathy interview, there would have been no way that the participant would have known that her interviewee had such a profound interaction with the healthcare system at a young age as to warrant a mid-life career change. It may feel strange to probe so deeply into the user's nuances and complexities, but it is the duty of the designer to engage the user genuinely and to learn raw insights that will later evolve into impactful innovations.

2.2.4 The Data Behind Design Thinking

Empathy interviews are chances to create data points from real users. The data produced during the empathy stage could be from interviews, phone calls, user journals, shadowing the user, photo journals, or any other mean of learning the user's perspective. From these insights, a designer would likely categorize the findings, seek patterns in the data, and discern insights from the observations. A simple empathy categorization method is an empathy map (Stanford D School 2010) (Fig. 2.2).

The goal of an empathy map is to distill the needs of a user in a routine and systematic way. An empathy map breaks down an empathy interview into four key groupings: the user's thoughts and beliefs, feelings and emotions, actions and behaviors, or quotes and defining words. If a designer repeats this process multiple times with different users, patterns emerge among the collective body of interviewees giving rise to a growing need.

When finding patterns in the data, it is important to note than not all users are the same. People have vastly different needs and lifestyles leading to a dichotomy in the design community known as extremes and mainstreams (Design Kit 2019b). Extreme users are the minority who inhabit disparate opinions towards the project at hand. Mainstream users are the majority who carry the popular opinion towards the project at hand. Empathy is useful to uncover the varying needs and desires for different users, especially extreme users. In global health, an appreciation for the vastly differing needs of users enables more tailored innovations. In the Ebola case previously discussed, the fear of ghostly health workers wearing PPE may have been the opinion held by extreme users, but these extreme users may also have been the

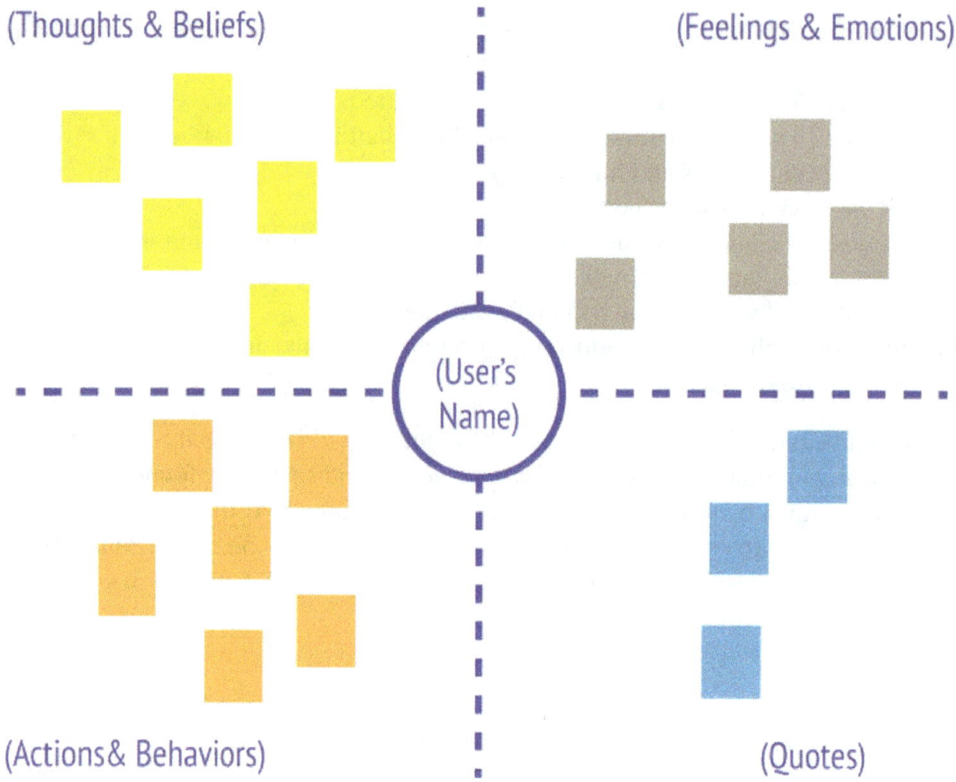

Fig. 2.2 Empathy map. Colored rectangles represent sticky notes

group disproportionately transmitting the disease. In this case, a tailored innovation for the extreme users would be most impactful.

2.2.5 Problem Definition and Problem Reframing

Following empathy, participants were introduced to problem definition and problem reframing. In design thinking communities, the problem definition and problem reframe are notoriously challenging. Defining a problem involves brutal honesty with oneself regarding the purpose of the design thinking project and the challenges facing the user. Sometimes designers believe they know the challenges facing the user without ever consulting the user through empathy. This leads to blind designing where products are built that completely miss the mark and do not address the user's true need. To avoid this horrendous mistake, always define the problem facing the user honestly.

Reframing the problem is equally challenging. To reframe the problem, one needs to know the systems that generate the problem and have the perspective to identify the root cause of the challenge.

Example: Creating a Music Ecosystem

An example of a problem definition and problem reframe is Apple's entrance into the music industry. When Apple decided to enter the music industry, the logical next step in product development should have been to create a device that would compete with the Sony Walkman. This device, by all means, would have built upon Apple's expertise in the computer industry and have been a smaller, more portable Macintosh.

Apple did create the iPod, which performed much like a smaller computer with the ability to play MP3 songs; however, during the process of creating the iPod, Apple reframed the problem users faced with the music industry. During the time when Apple was creating the iPod, the music industry was having challenges with illegal music piracy (Silverthorne 2004). Consumers could freely download music from illegal websites and store these songs on devices for listening. Downloading music was not the issue for consumers; finding quality music and sharing this music with friends was an issue. During the process of creating the iPod, Apple also created iTunes, a platform that would become the largest in its time. Apple addressed the challenge of finding quality music so well that people would pay to download songs from iTunes even though free piracy services still existed. By reframing the problem from listening to music to finding and sharing music, Apple created a product and a platform that would dominate the music industry for years to come (IIT Institute of Design 2009).

2.2.6 Bold Innovations

As the final didactic teaching moment for participants of the KKU Datathon workshop, a framework was presented to help participants categorize innovations and to be open to bold, groundbreaking innovations. This framework categorized innovations as either step, jump, or leap (Fig. 2.3).

Often, ideas that are seen as bold innovations are simply not as disruptive as one might think. These ideas are predictable and are the obvious iteration. These are step innovations. Jump innovations are where the starting point for the innovation is known, but the endpoint for the innovation is not. A jump innovation may start with a clearly defined problem but end with a solution that was unexpected. The last category is the leap innovation. These innovations are groundbreaking in that once they are introduced, they alter the landscape and workflows of their field forever. A leap innovation example is Airbnb where after its introduction, all around the world people changed how they viewed spaces in their home, travel, and the definition of a hotel (Thompson 2018).

Leap innovations are similar to Clayton Christensen's popularized term—disruptive innovation (Christensen 2012). These groundbreaking innovations are hard to materialize and often result in failure. Regardless of the risk involved in leap innovations, truly great companies, researchers, and entrepreneurs must take leap innovations and have a willingness for success and failure alike. Creative companies are

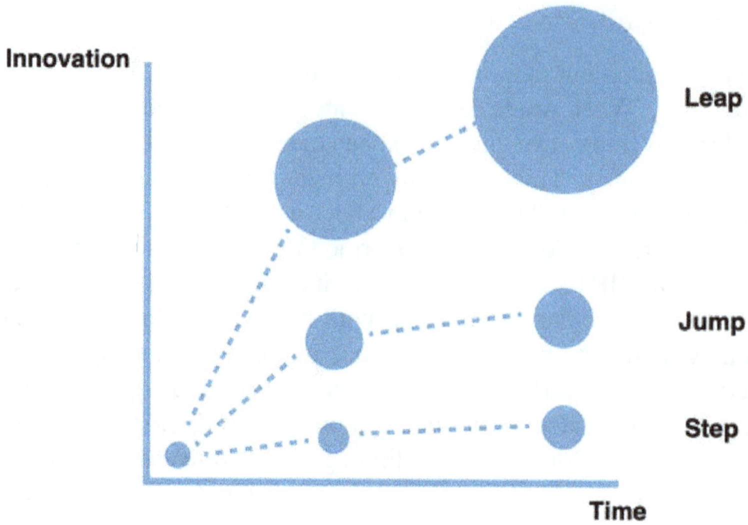

Fig. 2.3 Step, jump, leap

known for encouraging leap innovations by rewarding failure (Acton 2017; Bodwell 2019). Incentivizing failure loosens the shackles of conservative innovation from teams and enables bolder ideas. During the KKU Datathon workshop, a preference for leap innovation was stated as this opened participants to opportunities and realities with the greatest potential impact.

2.3 Part II: Application of Design Thinking

At this point in the KKU Datathon workshop, participants learned the skills needed to begin working through their respective design challenge in frailty. For this phase of the workshop, we use the five stages of the design thinking process as put forth by the Stanford D-School (Stanford D School 2010). Using the five stages, we helped participants indulge their creative capacity and apply skills learned earlier to develop new innovations. Participants began the design thinking journey by familiarizing themselves with the design briefs. A design brief is a short and concisely worded framing of the problem that needs to be addressed. Design briefs provide context and direct the designer where to begin the innovation journey (Open Design Kit 2018). A properly constructed design brief acts as the first stepping stone in the design thinking journey. Below are the design briefs that were supplied for participants of the KKU Datathon workshop.

2.3.1 *The Design Brief*

Three design briefs were provided for participants:

1. Preventative Care Measures Among the Pre-frail.
2. Addressing Challenges Among the Actively Frail.
3. Quality of Life Among Frail Individuals with Declining Health.

These three cases each captured different stages of life for the particular fictitious user, Joy Susan, who had unique needs and aspirations. All three cases pulled upon central themes and challenges among the elderly and all three cases needed thoughtful innovations to address the challenge presented.

2.3.2 *First Case—Preventative Care Measures Among the Pre-frail*

The first case introduced a fictitious, elderly woman, Joy Susan, who was 71 years of age, married, and overall decently sound in mind and body, but was beginning to show signs of decline. Joy Susan was pre-frail. She was on the cusp of showing the frailty phenotype—physical weakness, slow walking, low physical activity, low energy, weight loss—but was only partially frail. Joy Susan was experiencing functional decline and she and her husband were both concerned.

2.3.3 *Second Case—Addressing Challenges Among the Actively Frail*

The second case introduced Joy Susan as an actively frail older woman who was contemplating an upcoming surgery. As a frail individual, she had added concern for complications following her surgery. Her husband was especially concerned about the potential for delirium since he heard a doctor say this may be a complication (Verloo et al. 2016). Joy was actively weighing the possible benefits of her surgery against the potential complications that could result.

2.3.4 *Third Case—Quality of Life Among Frail Individuals with Declining Health*

The last case introduced a challenging design space where Joy Susan neared the end of her life. Joy had been severely frail for quite some time and her health outlook was not favorable. At this moment, Joy had difficulties embracing her situation,

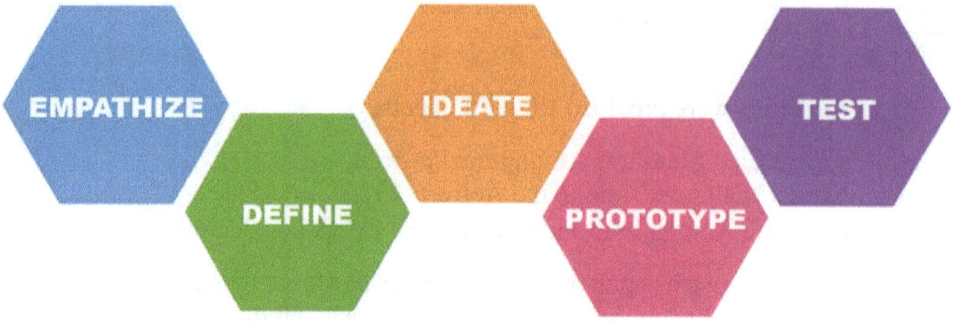

Fig. 2.4 The design thinking process

the physician had difficulties conversing to Joy about her options, and her husband struggled to embrace Joy's situation as well.

2.3.5 Beginning the Design Thinking Process

Each of the three design briefs posed a challenging problem with an unclear answer as to the best direction to follow. Especially for challenges such as those posed to Joy Susan where the immediate answer may not be known, design thinking is especially useful. By first uncovering Joy Susan's needs through empathy and then building from the empathy insights, teams had the chance to create profound new products and ideas. Participants started with empathy and continued through the full design thinking process (Stanford D School 2010) (Fig. 2.4):

1. Empathize
2. Define
3. Ideate
4. Prototype
5. Test.

2.3.6 Logistics

The original 25 participants were divided into teams of 8. Each team had a different design brief and worked through the following schedule with hands-on mentoring from the workshop leader. A PowerPoint highlighted directions for participants and a timer was used to keep the teams from lingering too long on any one part of the design process. Each portion of the below agenda is explained in further detail later on.

1. Empathize
   a. 10 min: 2 rounds of 3 min interviews with the remaining time spent writing down thoughts
2. Define
   a. 15 min: 3 min writing down personal insights, 3 min sharing insights, 9 min defining the point of view statement
3. Ideate
   a. 15 min: 6 min crafting the 'how might we' statement, 3 min personal ideation, 3 min group ideation, 3 min selecting the top idea
4. Prototype
   a. 10 min: all time spent building prototypes
5. Test
   a. 10 min: 3 min per team sharing their user's story, needs, aspirations, and the insightful innovation.

1. **Empathize**
   Within their teams, participants created pairs and interviewed each other about their particular design brief. The difficulty with this form of empathy was that Joy Susan was not present for individuals to question or interview. Rather, participants drew upon their relatives, interactions with elderly adults who had similar stories, or own opinions about how Joy Susan might feel with respect to each design brief. At the end of the Empathize section, Joy Susan became a much more real individual with desires and needs that were both complex and embedded within her relationship to her family, husband, job, and more.
2. **Define**
   The define stage was marked by teams sharing insights found through empathy interviews and then later defining the point of view (POV) statement (Rikke and Siang 2019). It was important that groups share their notes from empathy since the interviews were conducted within pairs and not all team members had the same conception of their Joy Susan. The difficult part of the Define section was creating the POV statement (Fig. 2.5).
   Using a prompt, teams each spent the next few minutes identifying the problem Joy Susan faced that they found to be most poignant. The POV statement needed

Joy Susan needs a way to ______________
(verb)

because ______________________________ .
(surprising insight)

Fig. 2.5 POV statement fill-in-the-blank

to have two components: (1) an action that Joy Susan had difficulties accomplishing and (2) a reason as to why this action was important to Joy Susan. The first part of the POV statement identified a challenge in Joy's life whereas the second half drew upon Joy's unique needs and aspirations. In general, teams needed help identifying a problem that needed to be accomplished without providing a solution as well. During the Define phase, no solutions were provided. Rather, only problems were shared and the reasons as to why the problems were pertinent to the user.

3. Ideate

During the Ideate phase, teams were finally able to start working through creative solutions to Joy's challenges. The Ideate phase was broken into two sections: (1) crafting a how might we (HMW) statement and (2) ideating around the HMW. A HMW statement is a launch pad for generating ideas. *How* opens the team to the reality that solving Joy's challenge is possible. *Might* shows the team that it is alright to fail during this process. *We* shows the team that this process is inclusive and collaborative (Google 2018). Crafting a proper HMW statement involves providing just the right amount of specificity to hint as to the direction for innovation while building upon the user's needs and aspirations. For instance, an HMW statement that is too narrowly focused is as follows:

1. *How might we* provide digital resources in mobile format to guide Joy Susan through her pre-operative procedure
   This HMW statement provides a solution already to Joy's challenge with surgery: digital resources in mobile format. The HMW statement also does not tie to any insights about Joy Susan. Lastly, this HMW statement does not enable the participant to generate that many ideas due to its narrow focus. The following HMW statement is too broad:
2. *How might we* lessen Joy's fears?
   Why is Joy afraid? How do we know where to target our ideas and innovations? This HMW statement is so broad that a designer would not know where to begin in ideating solutions.
3. *How might we* engage Joy's family through the pre-operative journey to lessen Joy's fears about family relations falling apart?
   This HMW statement identifies a direction for the innovation—engaging family pre-operatively—and provides an insight to ground ideas that are provided—lessen Joy's fears about family relations falling apart. The HMW statement is not too broad and it is not too narrow. It leads designers to the sweet-spot of ideation.
   After crafting the right HMW statement, teams used sticky notes to write down ideas that could solve the problem and then shared these ideas as a group. Three minutes were provided for personal ideation since solo-ideation leads to greater quantity of ideas produced. Then, group ideation followed where participants shared ideas together.

4. **Prototype**

Once teams had selected their desired solution for Joy's challenges, teams were directed to prototype their idea. The only supplies provided for teams were markers, sticky notes, and easel-pads. Teams created paper prototypes—drawings or sketches—or acted out their prototypes to convey the innovation. The key to a successful prototype is the ability to create something tangible that can be used or engaged with by a real user.

5. **Test**

The final step in the design process and the workshop was to test the prototypes with each other. The form of testing used during the workshop was a design critique (David and Yu 2017). Each team had 3 min to present Joy's challenge, her desires and needs, and then the solution created to solve Joy's problem. Following the presentation, other teams provided feedback that would be incorporated into future versions of the prototype.

2.3.7 The End Result: Khon Kaen University Datathon Workshop 2018 Prototypes

Pre-frail: Full Recovery

The first team was tasked with helping Joy overcome her challenges as a pre-frail individual who was sensing a looming health decline. The team identified the potential disconnect between Joy and her husband, Sam, that would arise as Joy's health declined. Who would take care of Joy if Sam wished to go outside? How could Joy stay connected with Sam as her health declined? The proposed solution: *Full Recovery*, a preventative home visit and consulting service to deter health decline and falls among the elderly. *Full Recovery* works to assess Joy's home environment before she becomes actively frail to see if there are features of her house or her living situation that could pose potential threats to her as she ages. *Full Recovery* would then create a list of activities that Joy performs at home for the physician to see. This way, the physician has a better sense of what is valued by Joy and how Joy's healthy decline is manifesting itself in activities that matter to her. If Joy enjoys gardening, the physician would know this and be able to see if Joy's treatment plan enables more gardening in the future.

Actively frail: Re-happy

The second team was tasked with designing an innovation for an actively frail Joy who was contemplating an upcoming surgery. The team identified the challenges of depression among the elderly, especially following surgery due to prolonged bedridden periods as a particular challenge for Joy. This team's solution was *Re-Happy*, a virtual reality system to allow Joy to explore and travel within a virtual world during the course of her recovery. The game would enable Joy to travel to new places, complete challenges, and also track her recovery. This innovation was addressed Joy's desire to stay immersed in the outdoors, which was a source of happiness for Joy, even during her prolonged bedridden recovery process.

End of Life: FulFill

The third and final team redesigned the end of life experience for Joy. This team tackled the communication breakdown that would occur for Joy through a platform called *FulFill*, which was a data-gathering platform to capture Joy's preferences and updated the family and physicians on Joy's desired course of action. The platform provided navigable care options and showed possible end of life scenarios for Joy to decide how she wanted her treatment to proceed. This team tapped into the difficulty Joy would experience in understanding her care options at such an advanced age and also relaying her care desires with her family. *FulFill* was a platform for sharing health information and end of life decisions that could be digested by both family members and physicians alike.

2.4 Conclusion

In global health, design thinking can be applied to ensure that resources, products, and services address the true needs of the people they intend to serve. By understanding the needs of the target population and testing proposed solutions rapidly, design thinking teams can avoid common pitfalls when delivering on a new innovation. Whether the challenge is to implement an intervention in a small community or devise a population level digital solution, innovators can benefit from the principles and application of design thinking. During the brief KKU Datathon workshop on design thinking in global health, participants formed teams and quickly exercised their creative capacity by delivering three tailored innovations to address challenges among frail older adults. Most certainly, these three innovations as they were delivered at the KKU Datathon workshop were not finalized, ready to implement, nor sustainable. One quick entanglement with the design thinking process did not bring about finalized products, but it most certainly guided the teams where the solution might be that would address a true user need. For readers who are curious about bringing products to market and building sustainable startups, an entrepreneurial guidebook will help. For readers looking to build creative capacity in their organization and lead teams that produce insightful innovations, design thinking is the avenue to pursue.

References

Acton, A. (2017). The most creative companies are the ones that celebrate failure. Here's how to do it effectively. Retrieved May 20, 2019, from Inc. website: https://www.inc.com/annabel-acton/stop-talking-about-celebrating-failure-and-start-doing-it-with-these-4-ideas.html.

Bodwell, L. (2019). 3 non-basic ways for incentivizing employees to innovate. Retrieved May 20, 2019, from Forbes website: https://www.forbes.com/sites/lisabodell/2019/01/31/incentivize-employees-to-innovate-from-futurethink/#7c7b93963d11.

Christensen, C. (2012). Disruptive innovation. Retrieved May 20, 2019, from Clayton Christensen website: http://claytonchristensen.com/key-concepts/.

Crossan, A. (2015). For Ebola patients, a way to see the faces of those helping. Retrieved May 20, 2019, from PRI's The World website: https://www.pri.org/stories/2015-04-07/ebola-patients-way-see-faces-those-helping.

Dam, R., & Siang, T. (2019). Stage 2 in the design thinking process: Define the problem and interpret the results. Retrieved June 13, 2019, from Interaction Design Foundation website: https://www.interaction-design.org/literature/article/stage-2-in-the-design-thinking-process-define-the-problem-and-interpret-the-results.

Design Kit. (2019a). The five whys. Retrieved May 20, 2019, from IDEO website: http://www.designkit.org/methods/66.

Design Kit. (2019b). Extremes and mainstreams. Retrieved May 20, 2019, from IDEO website: http://www.designkit.org/methods/45.

Ensrud, K. E., et al. (2007). Frailty and risk of falls, fracture, and mortality in older women: The study of osteoporotic fractures. *Journals of Gerontology—Series A Biological Sciences and Medical Sciences*. https://doi.org/10.1093/gerona/62.7.744.

Google. (2018). The 'how might we' note taking method. Design Sprints. https://designsprintkit.withgoogle.com/methodology/phase1-understand/how-might-we.

Heffernan, M. B. (2019). The PPE portrait project. Retrieved May 20, 2019, from http://www.marybethheffernan.com/about-the-ppe-portrait-project/.

IDEO U. (2019). Design thinking: A process for creative problem solving. Retrieved May 20, 2019, from IDEO U website: https://www.ideou.com/pages/design-thinking.

IDEO. (2019). Design thinking defined. Retrieved May 20, 2019, from IDEO website: https://designthinking.ideo.com/.

IIT Institute of Design. (2009). Patrick Whitney on the value of abstracting design problems. Vimeo. https://vimeo.com/5750600.

Jones, C. (1992). *Design methods*. Wiley.

Kelley, T., & Kelly, D. (2019). Creative confidence. Retrieved May 20, 2019, from IDEO website: https://www.creativeconfidence.com.

Nussbaum, B. (2011). Design thinking is a failed experiment. So what's next? Retrieved May 20, 2019, from https://www.fastcompany.com/1663558/design-thinking-is-a-failed-experiment-so-whats-next.

Open Design Kit. (2018). Design brief. Retrieved May 20, 2019, from Open Design Kit website: http://opendesignkit.org/methods/design-brief/.

Reeves, K., et al. (2008). *Qualitative research methodologies: Ethnography*. https://doi.org/10.1136/bmj.a1020.

Royere, D., & Yu, S. (2017). A practical guide to running effective design critiques. Retrieved June 13, 2019, from Medium website: https://medium.com/@suelynyu/a-practical-guide-to-running-effective-design-critiques-c6e8166c9eb0.

Silverthorne, S. (2004). Is iTunes the answer to music piracy? Retrieved May 20, 2019, from HBS Working Knowledge website: https://hbswk.hbs.edu/archive/is-itunes-the-answer-to-music-piracy.

Stanford D School. (2010). Empathy map. Retrieved May 20, 2019, from Stanford D School Old website: https://dschool-old.stanford.edu/groups/k12/wiki/3d994/empathy_map.html.

Stanford D School. (2010). An introduction to design thinking—Process guide. In *Hasso Plattner Institute of Design at Stanford University*. Retrieved from https://dschool-old.stanford.edu/sandbox/groups/designresources/wiki/36873/attachments/74b3d/ModeGuideBOOTCAMP2010L.pdf.

Thompson, D. (2018). Airbnb and the unintended consequences of "disruption." Retrieved May 20, 2019, from The Atlantic website: https://www.theatlantic.com/business/archive/2018/02/airbnb-hotels-disruption/553556/.

UNICEF. (2019). *UNICEF Democratic Republic of Congo Ebola Situation Report*.

Verloo, H., et al. (2016). Association between frailty and delirium in older adult patients discharged from hospital. *Clinical Interventions in Aging, 11*, 55–63.

Waters, H. (2011). Can innovation really be reduced to a process? Retrieved May 20, 2019, from Fast Company website: https://www.fastcompany.com/1664511/can-innovation-really-be-reduced-to-a-process.

WHO. (2018). Ageing and health. Retrieved March 19, 2019, from WHO News Room website: https://www.who.int/news-room/fact-sheets/detail/ageing-and-health.

WHO. (2019a). Ten threats to global health in 2019. Retrieved March 19, 2019, from https://www.who.int/emergencies/ten-threats-to-global-health-in-2019.

WHO. (2019b). Dementia Factsheet. Retrieved May 25, 2019, from https://www.who.int/en/news-room/fact-sheets/detail/dementia.

WHO Clinical Consortium on Healthy Ageing. (2016). WHO Clinical Consortium on Healthy Ageing topic focus: Frailty and intrinsic capacity. Retrieved from https://apps.who.int/iris/bitstream/handle/10665/272437/WHO-FWC-ALC-17.2-eng.pdf.

3

Developing Product Innovation in LMICs

Christopher Moses

Abstract In global health, innovation often comes from "outside-in": industrialized countries develop new drugs, devices, or services, and export them to low- and middle-income countries (LMICs) (Syed et al. in Global Health 9:36, 2013). Yet there is a growing recognition that there is real potential for "bi-directional flow of knowledge, ideas, skills and innovation" (Syed et al. 2013). To generate sustainable impact at scale, high-income countries should further encourage this local innovation capacity. One way to do so is to export more than just finished products to LMICs, but also the knowledge, processes, and cultural mindset that support repeated success in new product and service development.

Keywords Design thinking · Empathy · Outcome driven innovation · Agile Software Development · Product lifecycle

Learning Objectives

This chapter begins with an overview of core concepts in product innovation, then presents an innovation workshop. The goal of this chapter and its accompanying workshop is to provide teams with a set of fundamental concepts for thinking about new product development, as well as a detailed set of exercises whose output offers concrete steps for either increasing the chances of success for an existing product or service, or taking a brand new idea into the prototype phase. This workshop has been taught in multiple settings (corporate, academic, and startup) in both the United States and Thailand. By training teams in this way, we might best support nascent innovation capacity and help teams in LMICs bring more desirable, feasible, and viable innovations into their local communities, and potentially to the world at large.

C. Moses (✉)
Critical Data, Massachusetts Institute of Technology, 77 Massachusetts Avenue E25-505, Cambridge, MA 01239, USA
e-mail: cmoses@alum.mit.edu

3.1 Core Concepts in Product Innovation

There are many strategies high-income countries can leverage to best catalyze global health innovation in LMICs (National Academies of Sciences, Engineering, and Medicine 2017), but many of these approaches focus on technology investments. However, not all great innovations are technological in nature, and innovations in processes and implementation methods can have significant impact (Donaldson 2014). Interestingly, while the United States and other high-income countries are recognized for taking the lead in defining, refining, and systematizing innovation as a practice, their chief exports are often the products themselves rather than the less tangible, but critical knowledge and processes that enable repeated success in innovation. To build a common foundation for readers, we first review five core concepts in product innovation, and highlight frameworks that implement them. These frameworks are not mutually exclusive, and are in fact closely related in their approach to product innovation. Together, they can offer valuable points of view. These core concepts are (Table 3.1).

Table 3.1 The five core concepts of product innovation and their corresponding frameworks reviewed in this chapter

Core Concept	Framework
1. Conduct qualitative interviews to build empathy with users to better understand their unmet needs	Design Thinking (Brown 2009; Dam and Siang 2019)
2. Translate users' needs from high-level qualitative descriptions into standardized, testable statements to derive quantitative results that guide product development	Outcome Driven Innovation (Ulwick 2016)
3. Identify underlying assumptions about the user, their needs, or how the product or service will be implemented, then define a test plan to reduce risk and increase chances of success	Sense and Respond (Gothelf and Seiden 2017)
4. Test a new product or service with users as it's being built to better respond to changes in the user, their needs, and their environment	Agile Software Development (Beck et al. 2001; Koch 2011; Lucidchart Content Team 2017a)
5. Products have a lifecycle—a beginning, middle, and end—and there are important trade-offs to consider between product risk and operating cost over the life of the product	Think It, Build It, Ship It, Tweak It (Kniberg 2013)

3.2 Core Concept 1: Build Empathy with Users

In global health, those developing new products and services are often not the end beneficiaries of the innovation. As such, it is critical to deeply understand the target population as individuals to enable us to design more relevant solutions that better fit into their lives. Without building this empathy, we're more likely to miss important factors and apply misconceptions that could result in less useful products and failed implementations. As noted by Juma and Yee-Cheong (2005), "Creating appropriate products for low-resource settings requires not only a rethinking of what is considered a health technology, but also cross-disciplinary innovation and in-depth understanding of the particular needs of each country." Design Thinking is one popular approach to innovation with a foundation in building the empathy necessary to understand our target audience:

> What's special about Design Thinking is that designers' work processes can help us systematically extract, teach, learn and apply these human-centered techniques to solve problems in a creative and innovative way – in our designs, in our businesses, in our countries, in our lives. (Dam and Siang 2019)

For more detail on how to build empathy with users through qualitative interviews, readers are referred to the chapter by Tony Gallanis in this book and to Tim Brown's capstone book (Brown 2009) on Design Thinking.

3.3 Core Concept 2: Define Standardized User Need Statements

Spending time empathizing with users enables the designer to formulate the user's problems and goals in a user-centric way. These user need statements, also called problem statements or point-of-view statements, capture what a user is trying to get done and why. They can be defined in various formats (Gibbons 2019; Dam and Siang 2019; Barry 2010), and can help direct the ideation process when brainstorming solutions. For example:

> Carolyn, a frail retiree recovering from knee surgery, needs to learn and practice mobility exercises so that she can quickly return to her normal daily activities that really matter to her.

In his book, Jobs to be Done (Ulwick 2016), business consultant Anthony Ulwick proposed an alternative format for need statements as well as a process to enable teams to more exhaustively define, prioritize, and test which user needs are most significant and ripe with opportunity for innovation. His process, called Outcome Driven Innovation, focuses on better understanding what "job" a user is trying to get done, and how users measure the value of a solution they might use when getting that job done.

Given the user defined above, Carolyn's "job" is to recover from surgery. There are many solutions that might help her get that job done. Some solutions are better than others. But how do we know? We must understand how our users measure value. According to Ulwick, the way we do that is by understanding our users' *desired outcomes.* These tell us how our users gauge to what extent a solution helps them get their job done. For Carolyn, she might value the speed at which she recovers, her level of pain, and the extent of knee mobility she regains after surgery and physical therapy. Desired outcomes like these are uncovered during the course of empathizing with users, such as in user interviews.

3.4 Core Concept 3: Identify and Test Underlying Assumptions

New product innovation benefits from a diversity of input and feedback. We might think new discoveries and novel products are the result of the lone genius tinkering away in his or her laboratory or office, but more commonly innovation is the result of cross-disciplinary teams working together to achieve a common goal. This is perhaps even more prevalent in the global health context, where a multi-faceted and synchronized approach is crucial for successful implementation. This diversity is crucial for uncovering assumptions made by the innovation team.

Akin to testing a scientific theory, assumptions should be formulated into questions or hypotheses statements, then tested to validate or invalidate what the team is building or believes to be true. These hypotheses might be about the innovation itself (e.g. technical assumptions), about the users (e.g. who the users are or what they need), or about how the innovation might be built or implemented. For instance:

- Are we solving the right problem for our users?
- Do we have the right solution to those problems?
- How can we implement our solution to best reach our users?
- Can our solution be built? Does it depend on new science or new technology?
- Can our solution be sustainably financed, and sustainably fixed when it breaks?

One way to test whether or not the right problem has been identified is to rigorously uncover and test users' desired outcomes, as described in the previous section on the Outcome Driven Innovation framework. This and the other questions above represent risk that should be iteratively reduced over time to improve the chances of success. The next core concept offers one approach to addressing risk.

3.5 Core Concept 4: Adapt to Changes with Continuous Iteration

Most global health initiatives are static and follow the traditional, linear product development cycle. In software development, the traditional approach follows the Waterfall methodology, where requirements are fully specified upfront, the design is executed, then the software is finally built, tested, and shipped to users. While the Waterfall approach can be used successfully to deliver "clean" bug-free code and new features, it does a bad job in helping teams quickly respond to changes in the market, such as evolving user needs, or in managing the inherent uncertainty of the software development process itself (Lucidchart Content Team 2017b).

The Agile approach to software development, popularized by the publication of the *Manifesto for Agile Software Development* in 2001 (Beck et al. 2001), was developed in response to the weaknesses of the heavier, more planned Waterfall approach. Several methods implementing Agile principles have been developed over the years, and include Scrum, Kanban, and Extreme Programming (XP) (Lucidchart Content Team 2017a). In general, Agile principles value experimentation and responding to change over following a strict product plan. This helps minimize sunk costs from over-planning or from building too much before testing the product with target users (Koch 2011).

If possible, teams should plan their product development in such a way that the product is developed in steps, where each step offers an incremental increase in value to the user and can be tested. In this way, the build process for each step will be drastically shorter than the build process for the entire finished product. Shorter build times enable teams to test those scoped-down products directly with stakeholders or end users, which provides a vital source of feedback to help guide the team. Regular testing can also help uncover assumptions that had not yet been identified. For instance, perhaps there are local government regulations that influence how a product or service can be sold or delivered, or there are unexpected social factors that affect last-mile implementation. Identifying these assumptions as early as possible helps reduce risk, and iterative product development is a key tool that enables these key insights to occur.

3.6 Core Concept 5: Products Have a Lifecycle

The final core concept and its framework are discussed in significant detail, as they provide a useful mental model to help teams better understand the entire innovation process, and allow us to tie together the previous four core concepts.

At the most basic level, products have four stages in their lifecycle: ideation, development, delivery to end users, and end-of-life or sunsetting, where products are taken off the market. Whereas Agile provides teams a set of values and practices to plan, develop, and deliver software during the development phase, it is helpful to

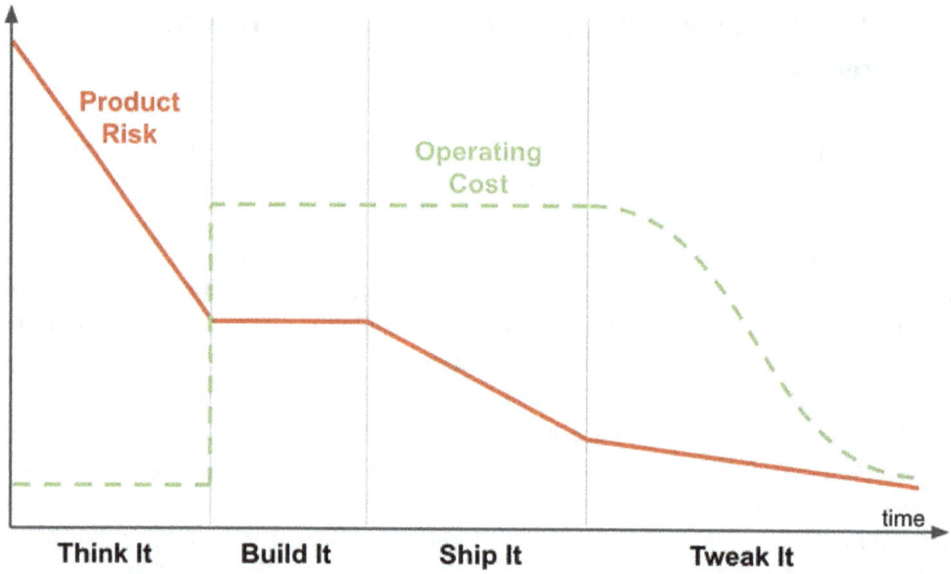

Fig. 3.1 In the Think It, Build It, Ship It, Tweak It framework, product risk is highest early in the product lifecycle, before the product has been built, tested, and shipped to users. However, the operating cost can be kept at its lowest during this early stage by committing only limited resources (e.g. a small team instead of a large team). Once product risk has been reduced through user testing and prototyping, more resources can be more safely committed (e.g. a larger team) as the product moves into the Build It stage

have a higher-level view of the entire product development lifecycle. This section provides an overview of the product lifecycle using the "Think It, Build It, Ship It, Tweak It" framework, developed by the company behind Spotify, the music app. Readers are referred to the original article (Kniberg 2013) for a more in-depth review of this framework. These four lifecycle stages help us understand important tradeoffs between product risk and operating cost over time.

3.6.1 Think It

The goal of the **Think It** stage is to provide the team evidence that their target users do in fact have a significant unmet need, and that the proposed solution might fulfill that need. The evidence must be compelling enough to further develop the product. If not, teams can save time and resources by shifting their efforts elsewhere. Teams should be able to answer by the end of this stage, "Are we building the right product?" To get at this answer, teams should start by defining all their assumptions, as well as criteria to help the team gauge whether or not the product is successful once launched. Basic assumptions that should be addressed include:

- Who is our user?

- What do they need?
- What value will this product provide them?
- What value will this product provide our team (or company) if it's successful?
- Can we build it?
- How will we acquire our users?

Examples of product success criteria include:

- User behavior measures, such as adoption and retention
- Technical measures, such as service uptime, total bugs, and bug severity
- Business measures, such as revenue, cost of customer acquisition or implementation, and length of sales or implementation cycle

Assumptions represent risk, which can be minimized by running tests, usually in the form of building and testing prototypes with potential users. Business and technical risks might also be reduced in this stage using other experiments, like measuring landing page conversion from a Google AdWords campaign that describes the software idea, or by building technical prototypes of the most challenging parts of the software architecture. In general, the more iterations tested, the better the final product (First Round Review 2018). There are a plethora of types of experiments teams can run. For a non-exhaustive list of examples, readers are referred to Jeff Sauro's writing on user research methods (Sauro 2014, 2015). This prototyping approach is extremely important in projects for global health initiatives. In a global health context, the product innovators are often not the same as the end users, even if the team is a local one. These differences in context can lead to a multitude of assumptions that could result in failure of the product or in its sustainable implementation.

Not all assumptions will be satisfactorily addressed during the **Think It** stage. It is a judgment call by the team for when to commit the resources to move forward with building the product. In addition, even if some evidence was acquired for certain assumptions, these tests often extend into the next lifecycle stages as the product is built and delivered. This is a different approach from many current global health initiatives, which rely on more traditional, linear development. The challenge is to strike a balance between enough good evidence to support the potential of a product and the speed of development. This ensures that the innovation cycle is faster and provides relevant, tangible, and timely interventions and products for the global health community.

The Innovation Workshop presented later in this chapter is designed to take place during the **Think It** stage, although it is applicable to the other stages as well. We come back to this point later in the chapter.

3.6.2 Build It

If the team agrees what's been prototyped is valuable enough to build, more resources are committed and the team enters the **Build It** stage. Operating costs increase as headcount goes up, but because the team hasn't yet shipped product to real users, they can't be sure they're further reducing product risk.

During this stage, it helps to narrow focus and prioritize efforts, as one team can't build everything, all at once. Instead, teams should prioritize work on the hardest, highest-risk assumptions first. A simple analogy is drug development—while it's easier to design the product packaging for a new drug (bottles, boxes), pharmaceutical companies instead focus first on testing whether or not a drug candidate can deliver on its target health outcome. Why develop the packaging if they can't build the drug? Teams should force-rank their assumptions defined in the Think It stage based on risk, with the greater-risk items having higher priorities. If two risks are gauged roughly equal, then the risk that is lower-effort to test should be prioritized higher to increase the speed at which teams can address these risks.

During the **Built It** stage, it's also important to develop the product from the start with a focus on quality: well-written code and robust, performant product components. However, this doesn't mean delivering the perfect product. The balance is in delivering a narrow product with the fewest possible features such that it delivers compelling value to the user, but built in a way that it won't catastrophically fail during usage. Once a small increment of working product is built, it's ready to be delivered to users.

3.6.3 Ship It

The **Ship It** stage is when teams start to roll out product to real users. To manage risk during software development, teams often rollout products in three phases of increasing penetration into the user base: alpha, beta, and generally available. This requires teams to listen to user feedback, and iteratively fix bugs while maintaining focus on achieving their previously defined product success criteria. Particular success criteria, like service uptime or customer satisfaction, can help identify whether or not there are new problems to address as more users adopt the product. While there are no standards for how many users to reach during each rollout phase, the rule of thumb is to generate sufficient evidence for the success criteria that the team can confidently rollout to more users.

3.6.4 *Tweak It*

If success criteria continue to be met, and any performance issues that arose during rollout are addressed, the product or feature has achieved general availability when all target users have it available for use. At this point, the feature moves into the **Tweak It** stage. In this stage, the product or feature might be iteratively improved upon, or simply moved into a maintenance mode and supported by only occasional bug fixes. The operating costs in this stage decrease over time as product developers shift their focus to other projects. Products only leave this stage if they're fully deprecated or sunset.

In this model of product development, the operating cost (the cost it takes to build the product) is lowest during the Think It stage: there might only be a small team (2–3 people) developing prototypes, after which a larger team is hired to develop the product in the Build It and Ship It stages. However, the product risk is highest during the Think It stage as the team is not yet sure if they're solving the right problem or have the right solution. While this sounds like a grave challenge, in reality this presents a great opportunity to learn as much as possible (to reduce product risk) while the costs are lowest (before significant funds have been invested). In this way, by prioritizing research and development on the highest-risk assumptions, teams can incrementally collect evidence that helps them either change course or end the project entirely.

3.7 Core Concepts Summary

These core concepts and their corresponding frameworks are not mutually exclusive, and are often used in tandem during product development (see graphic below). For example, qualitative user interviews provide the foundation for formulating user need statements. These user need statements can be re-written as outcome statements following the Outcome Driven Innovation framework, which can then be tested to provide more quantitative data to guide the team. Assumptions about the product, user, and implementation plan can then be systematically identified, and a research plan developed using the Sense and Respond model. Next, Agile practices like iterative development and regular user testing can help keep the product relevant and focused on meeting the users' needs identified earlier. Finally, the "Think It, Build It, Ship It, Tweak It" framework helps us keep in mind that upfront testing of our hypotheses is very cost-effective, and even after a product has been implemented with its target users, a long tail "Tweak It" phase is often necessary to continue adjusting the product so it continues to meet its users' needs over time (Fig. 3.2).

Each framework contributes valuable methods to the innovation process. But it can be difficult to reconcile them into a cohesive model of effective product innovation. Together, these core concepts and the accompanying workshop exercises presented below provide both a high-level mental model for successful product development,

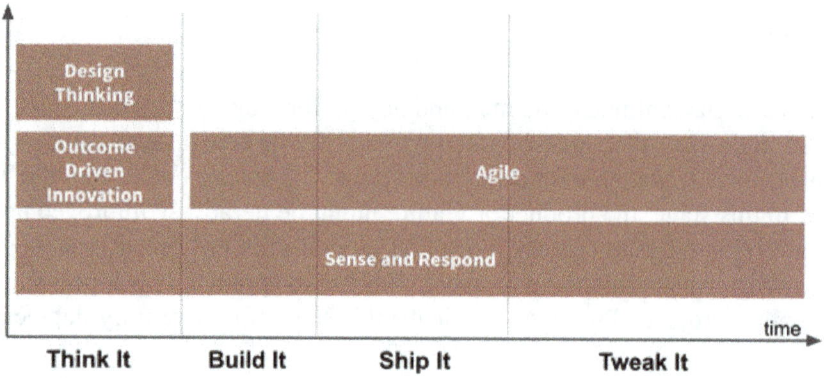

Fig. 3.2 The five frameworks fit together across the product lifecycle

as well as the tactical detail necessary to help teams implement innovation best practices. The goal is to enable teams to zoom out to understand where they are headed, then zoom back in to take measurable steps toward achieving their goals.

3.8 Innovation Workshop

In general, innovation is usually seen as more art than science, but in reality the innovation process can be broken down into concrete steps. By following a best practice innovation process, teams might both increase their chances of success as well as better repeat those accomplishments, thus creating a sustainable cycle of innovation. This workshop presents a set of eight exercises designed to generate discussion and produce a diverse set of ideas used to develop an actionable research plan for validating new product ideas.

During the workshop, teams identify target users, describe and prioritize their users' unmet needs, and then brainstorm features that might fulfill those needs. Next, teams identify any underlying assumptions they've made and then rank those assumptions by level of risk should their assumptions prove invalid. Finally, teams develop a user and market research plan for testing their highest-risk assumptions. The exercises are presented together as a single cohesive workshop, but each exercise can optionally take place individually over an extended period of time. The eight exercises are as follows:

1. Define your objective: 10 min
2. Identify target users: 5 min
3. Define users' needs: 10 min
4. Prioritize desired outcomes: 25 min
5. Brainstorm features: 35 min
6. Decide: 10 min
7. Identify assumptions: 15 min

8. Define the research plan: 10 min.

Each exercise is covered in more detail below, and in the accompanying workshop slides (Moses 2018). The workshop is designed for 2 hours of active time for exercises, with an additional hour for facilitator-led instruction to teach participants the five core concepts, for a total of 3 hours to complete the workshop. If there is more than one team participating in the workshop, there is an optional 20 minute exercise at the end of the workshop for teams to take turns presenting their results.

These exercises are not only for those interested in starting a commercial business or working in a large enterprise, but are equally as applicable for improving global health interventions. While the workshop is framed around product innovation, a "product" can be anything that meets a user's needs. Products need not have large user bases, nor do they need to be commercialized. A product might be physical, digital, or service-based. It can be proprietary or open source.

The workshop is designed to take place during the **Think It** stage of product development to give teams a foundation to kickoff new product innovation with the greatest chance of success. However, if teams have already progressed to prototyping, or have an existing product or service in use by their target population, they can still benefit from these exercises. Product functionality and product-market fit can always be improved. These exercises can direct more advanced teams to systematically assess what desired outcomes their product should be meeting, identify outstanding assumptions, and determine a research plan to test those assumptions.

The workshop is best conducted for a team of 5–7 participants. No prior entrepreneurial or product development experience is required. While more than one team can participate in the same workshop, each team is best served by a single dedicated, trained facilitator who is familiar with the instructions. Each team should have ample colored sticky notes, 5–7 sharpie markers, blank printer paper, and a large whiteboard for assembling their Outcome Map. For the Solution Sketches, it is helpful to use larger, 6 × 8 in. sticky notes. If that is not available, participants can fold a piece of printer paper in half. Slides for facilitating the workshop are provided in open-source format on Github (Moses 2018).

3.9 Workshop Output

The output of the workshop is organized into an outcome-based product roadmap, or Outcome Map. The Outcome Map is a simple visualization that combines a target user's desired outcomes, potential features that might meet those outcomes, assumptions about the user, product, or market, as well as ideas for testing those assumptions. It enables teams to collaboratively identify and refine a series of practical steps for effective product innovation (Fig. 3.3).

The Outcome Map is prioritized first by "Opportunity" (a measure of user's needs), then by risk. Teams may choose to prioritize the Outcome Map in other ways, such as by a measure of financial sustainability or technical feasibility. However, even if

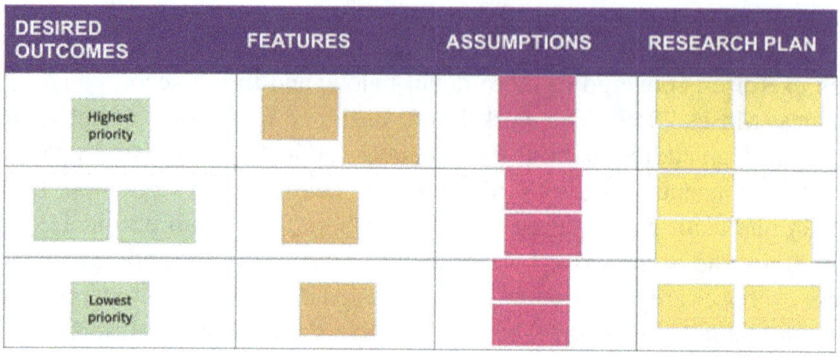

Fig. 3.3 The outcome-based product roadmap, or Outcome Map, that teams will develop in this workshop. The map can be assembled on a whiteboard or table using colored sticky notes

a product or feature is technically feasible, it might not be financially sustainable if there is not strong demand, i.e. if we do not target our users' significant unmet needs. For this reason, teams focus first on prioritizing by Opportunity to ensure they're meeting their user's greatest unmet needs.

To save time during the workshop and aid in presenting instructions to participants, it is helpful for facilitators to prepare the basic four-column structure of the Outcome Map on a whiteboard before the workshop begins. The facilitator might also provide a completed example Outcome Map to give participants better direction for how to define items within each column.

3.10 Workshop Scenario

The workshop provides participants the following shared scenario:

Laboratory studying interventions for treating frailty

Imagine we're working in a lab studying interventions to improve health outcomes for frail individuals, and preventing frailty among adults 65 years and older. Frail individuals have less ability to cope with acute stressor events like surgery or emergencies, which can lead to worse health outcomes than those who are not frail. Specifically, we've found that a group exercise program improves health outcomes, and we've published our results. A review article was recently published that cited our paper and backed up the evidence with additional articles supporting our findings. Our intervention is comprised of 5 upper- and lower-body exercises, done for 60 seconds each, 3 times per week, for 12 consecutive weeks. After reading an interesting article in Forbes describing significant business opportunities in this space, our principal investigator sets an objective to guide our team to productize our intervention:

> Launch a product or service that improves functional capacity and mobility for frail adults 65 years and older.

Table 3.2 Good and bad objective statements

Good objective statement	Bad objective statement
Launch a product or service that improves functional capacity and mobility for frail adults 65 years and older	Build a mobile app for seniors that delivers a workout plan that tailors 5 exercises for the user, and allows them to schedule and track their performance over time

3.11 Workshop Exercises

3.11.1 Exercise 1: Define Your Objective

Conventionally, in many companies product planning happens in a Waterfall fashion: the leader defines the vision and a 3–5 year product roadmap, and his or her leadership team translates that into each of their respective team's goals. The problem with this approach is that it doesn't take into account the inherent nonlinearity of product development, caused by the iterative nature of building, testing, and learning from users as well as changes in the market that might come from new regulations or the entry of a new competitor. Teams need a way to navigate these challenges without being constrained to any particular solution, but are provided enough guidance that they can remain focused on delivering their target user outcome. This can be accomplished with a well-defined Objective statement, which describes the outcome to be achieved but not how the team will achieve it (Gothelf and Seiden 2017) (Table 3.2).

3.11.2 Exercise 2: Identify Target Users

Imagine you were going to give a talk at a conference. When preparing, you might ask yourself, "Who is my audience?" Similarly, we need to understand our audience—our user when developing a product. In this workshop, we provide the following simplified user persona as part of our scenario:

Frail 85-year old after surgery

> I just had surgery and am returning home. Because I'm frail, I might have worse health outcomes. My goal is to recover as quickly as possible and to return to my previous state of health.

Participants should reference this user persona for the remaining exercises.

3.11.3 Exercise 3: Define Users' Needs

Participants are asked to brainstorm *desired outcome* statements for the target user persona defined above. For example, these statements might be:

Desired outcome statements

- Minimize the time it takes to recover from my surgery
- Minimize the likelihood I'm injured when exercising
- Maximize the amount of fat I lose when exercising

In reality, a user might have 100–200 desired outcomes, but for the purpose of this workshop, participants are asked to generate as many as they can in 5 minutes. Facilitators are urged to read Ulwick's book (Ulwick 2016) for more detail on this methodology.

3.11.4 Exercise 4. Prioritize Desired Outcomes

In Outcome Driven Innovation, user need statements are assembled into a survey, which is then fielded to hundreds of target users to provide more quantitative evidence to help teams understand which needs are most unmet. This is achieved by asking survey respondents to rank on a Likert scale their level of agreement with two key questions for each desired outcome:

1. When [doing the job or activity], how **important** is it for you to [achieve desired outcome]?
2. When [doing the job or activity], how **satisfied** are you with the way you currently [achieve desired outcome]?

For instance:

1. When recovering from surgery, how **important** is it for you to recover quickly?
2. When recovering from surgery, how **satisfied** are you with how fast you're currently able to recover from surgery?

By aggregating responses to these two questions, teams can visualize each desired outcome as a coordinate in a two-dimensional plot of Importance vs. Satisfaction. Those desired outcomes that rank very important but very dissatisfied reveal key opportunities for innovation (Fig. 3.4).

In lieu of conducting a large survey to collect quantitative data on users' ratings of satisfaction and importance, we use a quicker, easier method during the workshop. First, facilitators ask teams to force rank the desired outcomes they brainstormed in order of estimated importance to the user, from high to low. The facilitator records the rank order of each outcome, then asks the team to re-order the outcomes by estimated user satisfaction, from low to high. By adding together these two rank orders, and using the importance rank to break any ties between two equal sums, teams

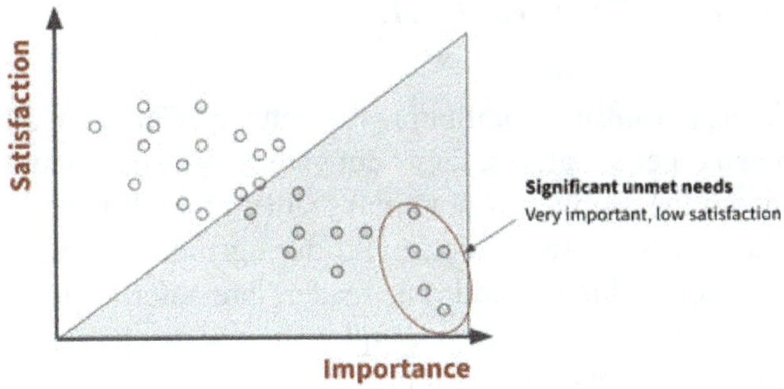

Fig. 3.4 A plot of desired outcome statements can reveal significant unmet needs

can approximate a relative "Opportunity Score." The desired outcome statements can now be placed on the Outcome Map in ascending order, where the smaller the Opportunity Score, the greater the users' unmet need, and the higher on the map the outcome will be placed. If they haven't already, facilitators ask the team to write the desired outcome statements on sticky notes and then place them on the left side of the Outcome Map in one vertical line.

At this stage, the participants have defined their user's needs and estimated the opportunity for innovation for each need based on how important and dissatisfied the user is in achieving that need. Next, we take these results and brainstorm features that might meet our user's needs.

3.11.5 Exercise 5: Brainstorm Features

What features will help our users meet their desired outcomes? Facilitators should remind participants to develop features that would help the user achieve their desired outcomes—not just the features they like. This section is broken down into three key exercises, adapted from the Design Sprint method developed at Google (Knapp et al. 2016), and described in more detail in the accompanying slide deck:

1. **Brain dump**: write down anything that comes to mind on a sheet of paper
2. **Crazy 8's**: rapid low-fidelity sketches of eight concepts, or a user flow of 1–2 concepts
3. **Solution Sketch**: more detailed sketch of a single concept.

Once the Solution Sketches are complete, facilitators ask teams to place them on the Outcome Map next to the desired outcomes they help achieve. If a feature achieves more than one desired outcome, then move that outcome statement into the same row.

3.11.6 Exercise 6: Decide

Time permitting, facilitators can setup a "Gallery Walk", where participants observe each other's features, then "dot vote" on the best ones. In this way, teams can narrow down the number of potential features they'll need to consider in the remainder of the workshop (and later, build during product development). This workshop does not detail this method, but readers are referred to Chapter 10 in the Sprint book (Knapp et al. 2016) for an explanation of this process. In this workshop, participants simply present their Solution Sketches to team members and vote on which one or two designs to move forward with.

At this stage, teams have defined their user's needs and brainstormed potential solutions for the most significant unmet needs given their estimated Opportunity Scores. The result of this exercise is to build a shared understanding of other team members' Solution Sketches, and to decide which one or two designs will become the focus for the remainder of the workshop. For instance, if a team of five produces five Solution Sketches, the team will vote to move forward with only one or two of the designs. In this way, teams can focus their efforts for the remainder of the workshop, where they exhaustively identify their assumptions, prioritize those assumptions by risk, and outline a research plan to test these assumptions.

3.11.7 Exercise 7: Identify Assumptions

As a group, have participants discuss the risks associated with delivering their chosen design(s). These risks might include:

- What challenges could the team face during product development? During implementation?
- What must be true about:
  - Our users?
  - Our technology?
  - State or federal regulations and policy?
  - The business model? Market?

Participants record assumptions on sticky notes and place them on the whiteboard, then force rank each assumption by risk. To rank by risk, ask: "How bad would it be if we got that assumption wrong?" For example, if your feature relies on access to user data, can you feasibly gain access to this data, and if so, how? How bad would it be if the technical approach you planned to use to access this data didn't work? If access to user data is critical to the functioning of your application, then this is a high risk and should be prioritized towards the top of your list. If your team also planned on a particular revenue model, but have not yet tested it, then that presents another risk. However, in comparison to the technical risk of your product not functioning if your team is unable to access user data, then this revenue model risk would be prioritized lower. In this case, by addressing that particular technical risk first, at least your team would have a functioning product, and perhaps could find a new revenue model if the one originally planned did not work out.

3.11.8 Exercise 8: Define the Research Plan

There are a plethora of user, market, and product research methods available to the team to validate their assumptions. Participants are asked to write one experiment per sticky note to address each assumption on the whiteboard. While the details of these methods are out of the scope of this book and workshop, a number of methods are listed in the accompanying slide deck for this exercise (Moses 2018). For example, teams might need to better understand their users, and could decide to run an ethnographic study or diary study to learn more about how their target users work. If a team needs to learn more about their product offering, they might build technical prototypes to investigate technical feasibility, or design a clickable prototype of screens to test the usability of a new product workflow.

3.12 Workshop Wrap Up

By the end of the workshop, teams have assembled an outcome-based product roadmap, or Outcome Map. Potential solution ideas are prioritized by users' greatest unmet needs, and the research plan is prioritized by risk. At this point, teams are still in the Think It stage of product development. Armed with a research plan, teams have greater direction for what to do next. However, facilitators should caution participants to carefully consider how much research they conduct. While teams will never achieve zero risk, they should strive to collect enough evidence to confidently decide whether to end the project, pivot to a new idea, or move forward with product development of their proposed solution.

In this workshop, teams focused primarily on solving for users' unmet needs, but participants are urged to think more holistically about a few additional factors when designing real-world applications. To successfully launch a product, even for global health and grant-funded projects, teams should carefully consider all of the following factors (Gerber 2019):

- **Desirability**
  - What significant unmet needs do our users have?
- **Feasibility**
  - What assets do we have (people, data, skills)?
  - Can we build it?
  - How long will it take to build it?

- **Viability**
  - Can we find a group of users or sponsors willing to pay?
  - Does the revenue or sponsorship cover the cost to build, sell, and service this product?

For example, even if we were to identify a large market of potential users and employed a team capable of building and delivering the product, there is risk no one adopts it if the product doesn't solve the users' significant unmet needs. By weighing these considerations, teams can better prioritize what to build.

3.13 Summary

Innovation is not a linear path, and there is no one right way. However, we *can* break down the process into faster, lower-cost chunks and then thoughtfully reflect on the outcomes along the way. As taught in this chapter and workshop, it is valuable to identify all high-risk assumptions upfront, then design experiments to test potential critical failures early on in the product development process. The Outcome Map is never complete, and is best treated as a living document. Similarly, product development never ceases—that is, until the product has achieved its goals and it comes time to deprecate it.

Building local innovation capacity by encouraging and teaching innovation best practices is only part of the puzzle. During debriefs with workshop participants at the 2018 Khon Kaen University Datathon in Thailand, the author learned that a cultural shift is also a critical component of progress. This is perhaps the greatest difficulty for a team, organization, or society to accomplish. In medicine, cultural change can be at the root of implementation challenges for evidence-based medical practices, despite clear results of positive outcomes (Melnyk 2017; Best et al. 2013; Rice et al. 2018). The reasons might seem intractable: limited resources, competing priorities, the need for leadership support and training, hierarchical relationships, a culture of shame for failure of new initiatives, among other factors.

But there is hope. In Estonia, the small Baltic country in former-Soviet Union, half of its citizens did not have a telephone line 30 years ago, yet today Estonia represents one of the most digitally-advanced societies in the world (A.A.K. 2013). Toomas Hendrik Ilves, the fourth president of Estonia, has said that Estonia's success in technological innovation has not been so much about using new technologies, but about "shedding legacy thinking" (A.A.K. 2013).

By rethinking how high-income countries might best catalyze global health improvements, we might derive new, effective, low-cost approaches. Building local innovation capacity through transferring knowledge, processes, and encouraging a culture shift about risk taking and failure offers an alternative. Given the inherent difficulties of culture change, local innovation capacity might be further supported by training teams in strategies for organizational change management techniques

(Kotter and Schlesinger 2008; Kotter 2014), in addition to innovation best practices. As a global community, we are still learning how best to catalyze global health improvements. Skill building in innovation best practices and organizational change management offers an alternative, low-cost approach to driving global health improvement.

References

A.A.K. (2013). How did Estonia become a leader in technology? *The Economist*. Retrieved 3 July 2019.

Barry, M. (2010). *POV Madlibs*. Hasso Plattner Institute of Design at Stanford University. Retrieved 25 April 2019.

Beck, K, Grenning, J., Martin, R. C., Beedle, M., Highsmith, J., Mellor, S., van Bennekum, A., Hunt, A., Schwaber, K., Cockburn, A., Jeffries, R., Sutherland, J., Cunningham, W., Kern, J., Thomas, D., Fowler, M., Marick, B. (2001). Manifesto for Agile Software Development. Agile Alliance. Retrieved 15 Nov 2018.

Best, A., Saul, J., Willis, C. (2013). Doing the dance of culture change: Complexity, evidence and leadership. *HealthcarePapers, 13*(1).

Brown, T. (2009). *Change by design: How design thinking transforms organizations and inspires innovation*. HarperBusiness.

Dam, R., & Siang, T. (2019). What is design thinking and why is it so popular? Interaction Design Foundation. Retrieved 24 April 2019.

Dam, R., & Siang, T. (2019). Stage 2 in the design thinking process: Define the problem and interpret the results. Interaction Design Foundation. Retrieved 25 April 2019.

Donaldson, K. (2014). 5 innovations in global health: Maybe not what you were expecting. *D-Rev Blog*. Retrieved 3 July 2019.

First Round Review. Six steps to superior product prototyping: Lessons from an Apple and Oculus Engineer. Retrieved 15 Nov 2018.

Gerber, J. (2019). How to prototype a new business. IDEO U. Retrieved 3 July 2019.

Gibbons, S. (2019). User need statements: The 'define' stage in design thinking. Nielsen Norman Group. Retrieved 25 April 2019.

Gothelf, J., & Seiden, J. (2017). *Sense and respond: How successful organizations listen to customers and create new Product*. Harvard Business Review Press.

Juma, C., & Yee-Cheong, L. (2005). Reinventing global health: The role of science, technology, and innovation. *The Lancet, 365*(9464), 1105–1107.

Knapp, J., Zeratsky, J., & Kowitz, B. (2016). *Sprint: How to solve big problems and test new ideas in just five days*. Simon & Schuster.

Kniberg, H. (2013). How spotify builds products. Retrieved 15 Nov 2018.

Koch, A. (2011). Expert reference series of white papers: 12 advantages of Agile Software Development. Global Knowledge Training, LLC.

Kotter, J.P. (2014). *Accelerate: Building strategic agility for a faster-moving world*. Harvard Business Review Press.

Kotter, J. P., & Schlesinger, L. A. (2008). Choosing strategies for change. *Harvard Business Review*. Retrieved 3 July 2019.

Lucidchart Content Team. (2017a). What is Agile methodology? *Lucidchart Blog*. Retrieved 5 July 2019.

Lucidchart Content Team. (2017b). The pros and cons of Waterfall methodology. *Lucidchart Blog*. Retrieved 5 July 2019.

Melnyk, B. (2017). Culture eats strategy: Why nursing and other health professions haven't fully embraced evidence-based practice. Medscape. Retrieved 3 July 2019.

Moses, C. (2018). Innovation Workshop. Github repository: https://github.com/cmoses8626/innovation-workshop.

National Academies of Sciences, Engineering, and Medicine. (2017). Global health and the future role of the United States. In *Catalyzing innovation*. The National Academies Press.

Rice, H. E, Lou-Meda, R., Saxton, A. T., et al. (2018). Building a safety culture in global health: Lessons from Guatemala. BMJ Global Health **3**, e000630.

Sauro, J. (2014). 10 essential user experience methods. MeasuringU. Retrieved 25 April 2019.

Sauro, J. (2015). 5 types of qualitative methods. MeasuringU. Retrieved 25 April 2019.

Syed, S. B., Dadwal, V., Martin, G. (2013, August). Reverse innovation in global health systems: Towards global innovation flow. *Globalization and Health 9,* 36.

Ulwick, A. W. (2016). *Jobs to be done*. Idea Bite Press.

4

EHR Databases: Development and Use

Lucas Bulgarelli, Antonio Núñez-Reiz and Rodrigo Octavio Deliberato

Abstract This chapter presents information about the development and use of Electronic Health Record (EHR) Databases. There are petabytes of untapped research data hoarded within hospitals worldwide. There is enormous potential in the secondary analysis of this clinical data, leveraging data already collected in everyday medical practice, we could gain insight into the clinical decision-making process and it's impact on patient outcomes. In this chapter we outline a high-level overview of some of the important considerations when building clinical research databases.

Keywords Electronic health records · Disease repositories · Data mapping · Data pipeline · Deidentification

Learning Objectives
The main objectives include:

- Understand the differences between traditional disease information repositories and EHR databases, and why they are useful
- Review examples of current EHR clinical databases
- Learn the necessary steps to develop an EHR clinical database

4.1 Background

4.1.1 Introduction to Clinical Databases

Health care information has traditionally been presented in "disease repositories"—a listing of manually collected disease specific information, often stored as aggregate registries. More recently, clinical databases have been developed, resulting in new

L. Bulgarelli · R. O. Deliberato (✉)
Laboratory for Computational Physiology, Massachusetts Institute of Technology, CA, USA
e-mail: deliberato.rod@gmail.com

A. Núñez-Reiz
Servicio de Medicina Intensiva, Hospital Universitario Clínico San Carlos, Madrid, Spain

ways to present, understand, and use health care data. Databases are defined as sets of routinely collected information, organized so it can be easily accessed, manipulated, and updated. Different from disease repositories, these new clinical databases are characterized by heterogeneous patient-level data, automatically gathered from the EHRs. They include many high-resolution variables originating from a large number of patients, thus allowing researchers to study both clinical interactions and decisions for a wide range of disease processes.

Two important phenomena accelerated the evolution of traditional disease repositories into new clinical databases. The first one is the global adoption of EHRs, in which paper-based systems are transformed into digital ones. Although the primary purpose of EHRs is not data collection, their implementation allows health systems to automatically gather large amounts of data (Bailly et al. 2018). Recognizing the enormous potential of the secondary analysis of these data for initiatives from quality improvement to treatment personalization, health and research institutions have started to leverage these novel clinical databases. The second phenomenon that supported the development of clinical databases is the extraordinary expansion of computational power that allowed the development of the necessary infrastructure to store vast amounts of diverse data, and the capacity to process it in a reasonable timeframe. These events enabled the emergence of the field of data science and machine learning. This new knowledge has been made accessible to a large and global audience through new massive open online courses (MOOCs), spurring substantial interest in analysis of large amounts of health data and the opportunity to crowdsource new machine learning techniques through available open source programming tools. (Sanchez-Pinto et al. 2018).

4.1.2 Goals for Database Creation

The main goal of creating a healthcare database is to put clinical information in a format that can be intuitively explored and rapidly processed, allowing researchers to extract valuable knowledge from the data. In a traditional database, there are relational structures built into store the data which guarantee consistency of the relationships between its entities (e.g. between patient and hospital visit). These structures are commonly referred to as "data models", and consist of the definition of tables, fields, and requirements for that database. When developing such models, it is essential to capture meaningful representation of the concepts and processes we want to study. This can be a challenge in health care because there are many different actors, and faithfully representing their relationships is crucial to understand what is occurring and also to achieve relevant and reliable research conclusions. Another critical step when creating and maintaining a clinical database is incorporating data quality and security, so it can be appropriately and reliably used in secondary data analysis.

4.1.3 *Examples of Clinical Databases Worldwide*

4.1.3.1 Medical Information Mart for Intensive Care (MIMIC)

The **M**edical **I**nformation **M**art for **I**ntensive **C**are (MIMIC) (Johnson et al. 2016) is one of the most popular and widely used open access clinical databases worldwide. Launched in 2003, MIMIC originated from a partnership between the Massachusetts Institute of Technology (MIT) Laboratory for Computational Physiology, Philips Medical Systems, and Beth Israel Deaconess Medical Center, with funding from the National Institute of Biomedical Imaging and Bioengineering. It is currently in its third version and has de-identified data from 40,000 medical and surgical patients admitted to the Beth Israel Deaconess Medical Center (BIDMC). Originally created with the aim of leveraging machine learning in the healthcare setting to build advanced ICU patient monitoring and decision support systems, MIMIC's main goal is to improve the efficiency, accuracy, and timeliness of clinical decision-making for ICU patients.

MIMIC has been used for many clinical studies from independent researchers (Aboelsoud et al. 2018; Johnson et al. 2018; Komorowski et al. 2018; Sandfort et al. 2018; Serpa Neto et al. 2018; Waudby-Smith et al. 2018; Block et al. 2018; Collins et al. 2014; Computing NCfB 2018; Deliberato et al. 2018; Dernoncourt et al. 2017; Desautels et al. 2016; Desautels et al. 2017; Farhan et al. 2016; Feng et al. 2018; Fleurence et al. 2014; Ghassemi et al. 2014; Johnson et al. 2016). Since its first version, MIMIC allowed researchers to freely access the data, after registering, completing a preliminary course on human research, and abiding by a data use agreement to avoid the potential misuse of clinical data. This has been one of the main reasons for its popularity in the clinical research community, along with the enormous quantity of diverse information for all patients in MIMIC, making complex cross-evaluating studies feasible. Another important feature for researchers is that individual patient consent has been waived by BIDMC's Institutional Review Board, an essential and challenging prerequisite to allow for a clinical database to go public in the real world.

In addition to clinical data extracted from the EHR such as demographics, diagnoses, lab values, vital signs, events, and medications, there is a subset of patients with bedside monitor waveforms from ECG, EEG, and vital sign tracings that are stored in flat binary files with text header descriptors. MIMIC also maintains documentation of data structure and a public GitHub repository for researchers interested in working with the database. As result, new users can benefit from the work of others by accessing the available code, and are encouraged to contribute their own work, thereby strengthening and furthering the impact of MIMIC.

4.1.3.2 eICU Collaborative Research Database (eICU-CRD)

Another example of an open-access database is the eICU Collaborative Research Database (eICU-CRD) (Pollard et al. 2018). This project is derived from a critical care telehealth initiative by Philips® Healthcare. The eICU-CRD was made freely available by the same team as MIMIC and features a distinct patient pool originating from 208 ICUs across the U.S. from 2014 to 2015. As a result, MIMIC and eICU-CRD are independent yet complementary. Similar to MIMIC, the main objective of the project is to boost collaboration in secondary analysis of electronic health records, through the creation of openly available repositories.

4.1.3.3 Other Databases for Collaborative Research

There are other clinical databases that can be used for collaborative research, although access is more restricted, and data tend to be more general and less granular than the clinical information available in MIMIC or eICU-CRD. One example is PCORnet (Collins et al. 2014), a patient-centered clinical research project that aims to build a national research network, linked by a common data platform and embedded in clinical care delivery systems (Collins et al. 2014; Fleurence et al. 2014). This network aims to provide enough data for studies of rare or uncommon clinical entities, that have been difficult to conduct with the "classical" model. Medical record collections from over 60 million patients allow for large-scale observational and interventional trials to be accomplished more easily (Block et al. 2018). Access to the data can be requested through their web platform "Front Door" and is granted with a case-by-case policy depending on the project.

Other initiatives aim to create common data models, enabling the construction of multiple databases using a common ontology, so that data from each source means the same thing. The Observational Medical Outcomes Partnership (OMOP) and i2b2 have been established using this concept and aim to translate healthcare concepts to a common language in order to facilitate the sharing of meaningful data across the compatible databases. OMOP is managed by a network called Observational Health Data Science and Informatics (OHDSI), a multi-stakeholder, interdisciplinary collaborative network that spans over 600 million patients. A list of databases ported to their model can be found at their website (Observational Health Data Sciences and Informatics (OHDSI) 2018; OMOP CDM 2018). The i2b2 tranSMART Foundation (Computing NCfB. i2b2 (Informatics for Integrating Biology and the Bedside) 2018) is a member-driven non-profit foundation with an open-source/open-data strategy. It provides an open-source data model similar to OMOP, and a list of databases can be found at their website (Computing NCfB 2018). Both OMOP and i2b2 have open source software tools to manage and access the data, and a very active community of users with forums where relevant information and implementation tips can be found.

4.2 Exercise: Steps for Building an EHR Database for Research

4.2.1 *Putting Together the Right Team*

One of the most important steps at the start of any successful project is putting together the right team. Bringing together the range of skilled professionals with the required skills is essential when building an EHR database. One key role is that of a clinician with the knowledge to understand and decipher the highly specialized data collected in the EHR, especially because these data are often poorly organized within the EHR. Clinicians also have an important role in assessing the accuracy of the resulting database and working with data scientists to optimize its usability for targeted end-users.

Another critical member for the team is someone with substantial knowledge in data architecture, who can ensure consistency while modeling the highly complex data from EHRs. This person needs to work closely with the clinicians and data scientists to achieve a high quality, functional clinical database.

4.2.2 *The Six Steps to Building an EHR Database*

Once the multidisciplinary team has been formed, the next step is familiarizing everyone with the steps for building the database. This is important because the process of building a clinical database is iterative and continuous, as developers work to guarantee data quality and security. The six main stages for developing a clinical database are summarized in Fig. 4.1.

4.2.2.1 Step 1: Access and Data Model

At the start of the project, it can be helpful to acquire some resources to help with some of the laborious tasks that are inherent in the process of building clinical databases. For instance, if the clinicians building the database work at the hospital where the data is generated, obtaining access to a real time copy of the EHR source database (Step 1, Fig. 4.1) can facilitate mapping. In this scenario, clinicians can use one of their current patients to search for the information that the data architects are trying to map in the EHR system. This helps locate the data to be mapped in the source database. It also helps validate the mapping, by comparing the current reported values after the information is found. This resource is extremely valuable in the assessment of data consistency, since most of the data found in these source databases are used only for maintenance of system functionalities and have no clinical value, thus confusing the mapping process. Although obtaining real time copy of databases may be useful, it can be difficult to do in resource limited settings. In such cases, looking for other

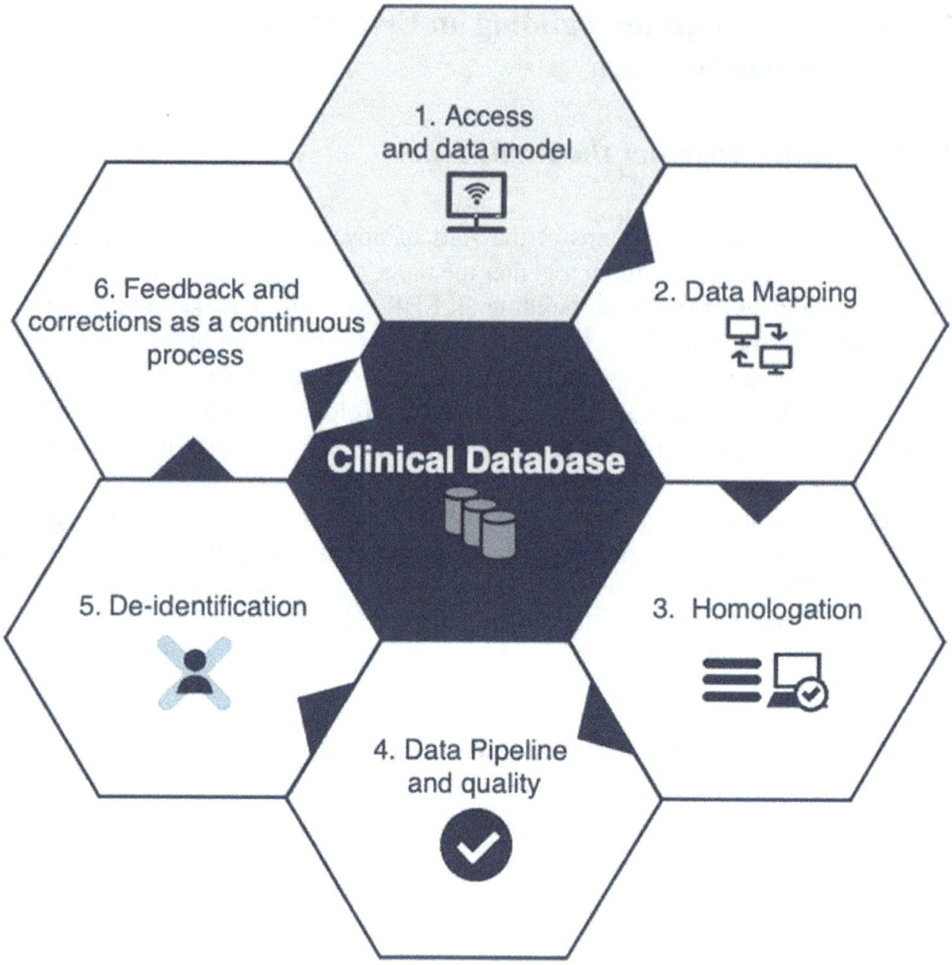

Fig. 4.1 Main stages for the process of clinical database development

ways using the available computational infrastructure in order to acquire the data in a faster time frame is recommended, as any highly available data is valuable in building the database and creating a data-driven environment.

In addition to working with a copy of the EHR source database, the database development team needs to combine their skills in data architecture with their knowledge about the targeted uses of the database in order to find a data model that would fit all the stakeholders' requirements (Step 1, Fig. 4.1). Balancing these needs is difficult, but critically important at this stage. While modeling all data to fit clinical or analytical mindsets might be desired, creating a model using high granularity and resolution data causes some limitations. Additionally, if conducting multicenter studies is one of the goals, the adoption of open-source health data models, or converging to a data model that can be used by prospective partners might be taken into consideration, as the use of common data models not only facilitates those studies, but also improves their reliability. It is important to emphasize that there is no ideal model and it is highly recommended to choose a common data model most likely to become part of the initiatives already in place in your institution, having an active voice in the process, and helping the community to decide the future direction of the model.

4.2.2.2 Data Mapping

With access to the EHR source database acquired and a data model determined, mapping the data will be main activity of both data architects and clinicians (Step 2, Fig. 4.1). This step is the longest in the process, so obtaining documentation from the source database will prove helpful and can shorten the time needed. Data architects will need to dive into the specifics of the source database, and work on the Extracting, Transform and Load (ETL) process, and fitting the data in the chosen data model. The clinicians' role in this stage is to help the data architects in finding the information in the source database, by browsing through the EHR system and identifying where data is stored. The clinicians will also need to validate the data whenever new information is added to the ETL, verifying if the information being stored corresponds with their actual clinical meaning, making each iteration of the data mapping more reliable and consistent. If the clinicians do not work in the source hospital, their expertise will be used to validate the iterations based on whether the given value for each variable is reasonable for its type.

4.2.2.3 Homologation

If the validation steps during the iterations of data mapping were performed well, the next step, homologation (Step 3, Fig. 4.1), will be short and only require small adjustments to the mapping. Homologation consists of checking to make sure all the mapped data are correct, and have not been corrupted during the ETL process, as a result of improper deletion or modification of information, inclusion of irrelevant and confounding data, and inaccurate verification of correct clinical meaning. During this process, some of the clinicians' current patients are randomly chosen and information from their latest stay is verified by comparing the information in their medical record to the mapped data. If real time access to the EHR source database was not obtained, this process can be more time consuming as the information from the randomly chosen patients needs to be adapted to the current conditions. If the clinicians on the database development team do not have access to the EHR system, they must homologate the records using their expert knowledge, as they did when validating the data mapping. It is very important that the database development team be thorough during the homologation process, as every piece of mapped information must be checked in order to guarantee the consistency of the data.

4.2.2.4 Data Pipeline and Quality

After completing the homologation process, the prototype of the database is essentially completed. The next step in the process is to establish the automatic input of the mapped data into a repository, by using a pipeline that assesses data quality (Step 4, Fig. 4.1). The pipeline is made up of sequentially executed computer tasks, scheduled and ordered according to desired intervals and availability of the source database, i.e. real-time or daily, in order to maintain the consistency of the data and the relationships between them. The last and most important task before the final incorporation of the data into the repository must be checking data quality, for example looking for values that differ significantly from current historical data, thereby preventing the inclusion of possibly corrupted data in studies utilizing the database.

4.2.2.5 De-identification

With the completion of the data pipeline, a usable database is in place. In order to have a clinical database that can be used by other researchers and applications, most institutions and governments require further development to comply with privacy policies and regulations. Additional steps, commonly referred to as de-identification, need to be included in the pipeline (Step 5, Fig. 4.1), in order to produce a database which complies with these requirements. For structured data, i.e. columns of a database, these methods rely on categorizing information, and then deleting or cryptographing the ones flagged as protected. For unstructured data, such as clinicians' notes, various methods of natural language processing are used, from simple regular expressions, that are pattern matching sequences, to sophisticated neural networks, ultimately trying to identify all protected information throughout the free text for deletion or cryptography (Neamatullah et al. 2008; Dernoncourt et al. 2017). These methods have been included in software and services (Amazon Comprehend Medical 2018) to assist healthcare institutions to comply with patient privacy policies.

4.2.2.6 Feedback and Correction to Continually Improve and Maintain the Database

After completing the first version of the database, the process is not over. It is essential to understand that constructing a database is a continuous process, relying on continual user feedback to improve and maintain the integrity of the information. The users will have important insights on what can be improved in future versions. The data architect who will be responsible for the maintenance of the database must continually monitor the source database and the pipeline for any possible data corruption. Additional data quality assessments with expert knowledge from clinicians are recommended, who can provide ongoing input regarding whether the data is being properly populated in the database. This can help detect problems in the EHR system, source database or inform directives on how clinicians input information in the EHR system.

References

Aboelsoud, M., Siddique, O., Morales, A., Seol, Y., & Al-Qadi, M. (2018). Early biliary drainage is associated with favourable outcomes in critically-ill patients with acute cholangitis. *Przeglad Gastroenterologiczny, 13*(1), 16–21.

Amazon Comprehend Medical. Retrieved from December 2018, from https://aws.amazon.com/comprehend/medical/.

Bailly, S., Meyfroidt, G., & Timsit, J. F. (2018). What's new ICU in 2050: Big data and machine learning. *Intensive Care Medicine, 44,* 1524–1527.

Block, J. P., Bailey, L. C., Gillman, M. W., Lunsford, D., Boone-Heinonen, J., Cleveland, L. P., et al. (2018). PCORnet antibiotics and childhood growth study: Process for cohort creation and cohort description. *Academic Pediatric, 18*(5), 569–576.

Collins, F. S., Hudson, K. L., Briggs, J. P., & Lauer, M. S. (2014). PCORnet: Turning a dream into reality. *Journal of the American Medical Informatics Association, 21*(4), 576–577.

Computing NCfB. (2018). i2b2 (Informatics for Integrating Biology and the Bedside). Retrieved October 2018, from https://www.i2b2.org.

Deliberato, R. O., Ko, S., Komorowski, M., de La Hoz Armengol, M. A., Frushicheva, M.P., & Raffa, J., et al. (2018, March). Severity of illness may misclassify critically ill obese patients. *Crit Care, 46*(3), 394–400.

Dernoncourt, F., Lee, J. Y., Uzuner, O., & Szolovitz, P. (2017). De-identification of patients notes with recurrent neural networks. *Journal of the American Medical Informatics Association, 24*(3), 596–606.

Desautels, T., Calvert, J., Hoffman, J., Jay, M., Kerem, Y., Shieh, L., et al. (2016). Prediction of sepsis in the intensive care unit with minimal electronic health record data: A machine learning approach. *JMIR Med Inform., 4*(3), e28.

Desautels, T., Das, R., Calvert, J., Trivedi, M., Summers, C., Wales, D. J., et al. (2017). Prediction of early unplanned intensive care unit readmission in a UK tertiary care hospital: A cross-sectional machine learning approach. *British Medical Journal Open, 7*(9), e017199.

Farhan, W., Wang, Z., Huang, Y., Wang, S., Wang, F., & Jiang, X. (2016). A predictive model for medical events based on contextual embedding of temporal sequences. *JMIR Medical Informatics, 4*(4), e39.

Feng, M., McSparron, J. I., Kien, D. T., Stone, D. J., Roberts, D. H., Schwartzstein, R. M., et al. (2018). Transthoracic echocardiography and mortality in sepsis: Analysis of the MIMIC-III database. *Intensive Care Medicine, 44*(6), 884–892.

Fleurence, R. L., Curtis, L. H., Califf, R. M., Platt, R., Selby, J. V., & Brown, J. S. (2014). Launching PCORnet, a national patient-centered clinical research network. *Journal of the American Medical Informatics Association, 21*(4), 578–582.

Ghassemi, M., Marshall, J., Singh, N., Stone, D. J., & Celi, L. A. (2014). Leveraging a critical care database: Selective serotonin reuptake inhibitor use prior to ICU admission is associated with increased hospital mortality. *Chest, 145*(4), 745–752.

Johnson, A. E., Pollard, T. J., Shen, L., Lehman, L. W., Feng, M., Ghassemi, M., et al. (2016). MIMIC-III, a freely accessible critical care database. *Scientific Data, 3,* 160035.

Johnson, A. E. W., Aboab, J., Raffa, J., Pollard, T. J., Deliberato, R. O., Celi, L. A., et al. (2018). A comparative analysis of sepsis identification methods in a electronic database. *Critical Care, 46*(4), 494–499.

Komorowski, M., Celi, L. A., Badawi, O., Gordon, A. C., Faisal, A. A. (2018, October 22). The artificial intelligence clinician learns optimal treatment strategies for sepsis in intensive care. Nat Med. [Epub ahead of print].

List of databases which have been converted to OMOP CDM. (2018). Retrieved October 2018, from http://www.ohdsi.org/web/wiki/doku.php?id=resources:2018_data_network.

Neamatullah, I., Douglas, M. M., Lehman, L. W., Reisner, A., Villarroel, M., Long, W. J., et al. (2008). Automated de-identification of free text medical records. *BMC Medical Informatics and Decision Making, 24*(8), 32.

Observational Health Data Sciences and Informatics (OHDSI) OMOP Common Data Model V5.0. Retrieved October 2018, from https://www.ohdsi.org.

Pollard, T. J., Johnson, A. E. W., Raffa, J. D., Celi, L. A., Mark, R. G., & Badawi, O. (2018). The eICU collaborative research database, a freely available multi-center database for critical care research. *Scientific Data, 5,* 180178.

Sanchez-Pinto, L. N., Luo, Y., Churpek, M. M. (2018, May 9). Big data and data science in critical care. *Chest* pii: S0012-3692(18)30725-6 [Epub ahead of print].

Sandfort, V., Johnson, A. E. W., Kunz, L. M., Vargas, J. D., Rosing, D. R. (2018). Prolonged elevated heart rate and 90-day survival in acutely Ill patients: Data from the MIMIC-III database. *Journal of Intensive Care Medicine,* 885066618756828.

Serpa Neto, A, Deliberato, R. O., Johnson, A. E. W., Bos, L. D., Amorim, P., Pereira, S. M., et al. (2018, October 5). Mechanical power of ventilation is associated with mortality in critically ill patients: an analysis of patients in two observational cohorts. Intensive Care Medicine [Epub ahead of print].

Waudby-Smith, I. E. R., Tran, N., Dubin, J. A., & Lee, J. (2018). Sentiment in nursing notes as an indicator of out-of-hospital mortality in intensive care patients. *PLoS ONE, 13*(6), e0198687.

5

Global Health Projects and Financial Resources

Katharine Morley, Michael Morley and Andrea Beratarrechea

Abstract Clinicians and engineers are improving medical practice and healthcare care delivery in low and middle-income countries (LMIC's) through research and innovation using data science and technology. One of the major barriers to translating their ideas into practice is the lack of financial resources. Without adequate funding, many of the critical issues regarding the development, implementation, and impact of technology innovations—including whether there is an actual improvement in clinical outcomes—cannot be adequately evaluated and addressed. While securing funding is a challenge for everyone, researchers and innovators in LMIC's often lack training and experience in proposal writing to support their work.

Keywords LMIC · Funding · Funding strategy · Grants · Implementation research · Grant writing · Funding · Research · Technology · Innovation

Learning Objectives

This chapter is designed to provide clinicians and engineers with information on how to develop an idea into a fundable proposal. We will focus on understanding why research is an important strategy in the development and implementation of digital innovations such as mHealth and artificial intelligence (AI) technologies, developing a problem statement and research question, understanding the components of a research proposal, and learning about funding sources and strategies. We use research as a framework for developing a funding proposal because funding opportunities for health care technology development and implementation often are centered around research. Even if you are not planning to seek funding for research,

K. Morley (✉)
Department of Medicine, Harvard Medical School, Massachusetts General Hospital, 15 Parkman Street, Boston, MA 02114, USA
e-mail: kemorley@mgh.harvard.edu

M. Morley
Ophthalmic Consultants of Boston, Harvard Medical School, Boston, MA, USA

A. Beratarrechea
Institute for Clinical Effectiveness and Health Policy (IECS), Buenos Aires, Argentina

National Scientific and Technical Research Council (CONICET), Buenos Aires, Argentina

the concepts in this chapter can be adapted to support the development of your idea for other types of funding opportunities. A "toolkit" with worksheets, guidelines, and additional reference materials is included to help you get started on your own funding proposal.

5.1 Background

5.1.1 Introduction

5.1.1.1 The Importance of Research in Digital Health Innovations

Why You Need to do Research in mHealth and Data Science

In order for any technology intervention to achieve an improvement in health, several requirements need to be met. The technology needs to be acceptable, usable, and feasible for the target population; a new technology cannot impact health unless people *actually* use it. This is especially true in LMIC's, where the culture and environment have a major effect on technology adoption. Research is necessary to determine the innovation's efficacy and impact—does it result in the desired clinical outcome in a controlled setting and how much of a true benefit is measurable? Finally, implementation research provides critical information about its use and effectiveness on a larger scale in real world situations (Tomlinson et al. 2013)

The number of mobile health apps is growing rapidly, and AI innovations are quickly being incorporated into powerful tools on smart phones. Many of these apps never make it past the pilot stage because they lack proof of usability and acceptability, clinical impact, and value (Roess 2017; Labrique et al. 2013). As a result, there are a plethora of incompletely developed apps of unclear value for clinicians and patients (Kuehn 2015). Research provides evidence for funders, investors and donors who all want to understand the potential impact and risks involved in all stages of technology innovation before making financial investments which are necessary for technology innovations to realize their promise of improving accessibility and quality of care in LMIC's (Kumar et al. 2013).

The Importance of Implementation Research

Successfully implementing a new process or innovation has many challenges. Understanding the technology, user, and context in which it will be deployed is critically important for success. Research focusing on implementation outcomes can help us understand why and how technology innovations are successful, or unsuccessful, so improvements can be made (Peters et al. 2013). For example, the developer of a smartphone app to help diabetics track blood sugar readings and diet may conduct

Table 5.1 General questions for technology research

• Why is/is not a new innovation an improvement? For whom? In what context?
• What are the barriers and facilitators for technology adoption?
• What new knowledge can we learn from large databases of information?
• How can we successfully implement a new process using a technology innovation?

Table 5.2 General concepts for developing a research proposal

Pay meticulous attention to details
Thoughtful organization
Good leadership and communication
Use a high level of scientific rigor

a qualitative research study using interviews and focus groups to identify facilitators and barriers for using the app. Studying these challenges and gaps is an important opportunity for maximizing the probability of a successful and sustainable innovation.

Pilot studies provide the opportunity for preliminary evaluation and are helpful before scaling up an intervention. They often reveal a myriad of adoption and feasibility issues and unintended consequences. Keeping with the example of a smartphone app for diabetics, a simple mixed methods pilot study looking at adoption might collect quantitative outcomes like the number and characteristics of users who stopped using the app within the first month, and then collecting feedback about why they did or did not continue. This information guides subsequent revisions in the technology and the way it is used, laying the foundation for rigorous research to demonstrate effectiveness of the innovation in a larger population.

5.1.1.2 Develop Your mHealth or Data Science Research Project

Going from an Idea to a Real Project

Ideas are where research and innovation start—but transforming an idea into a useful product requires effort, planning, and collaboration. In most cases, it requires funding as well. In this section, we present some general concepts for developing a research proposal and how it can be used as a framework for writing a funding proposal (Table 5.1). The general concepts for developing a research proposal, summed up in Table 5.2, are easy to understand. Applying these principles from the beginning is necessary for success.

Developing Your Research Question

Formally defining your research question is the foundation for any good research proposal. It clarifies and crystallizes the problem you want to address, and how you intend to address it. Importantly, it determines the study design, outcome measures, and analysis methodology you need to use. A good research question is clear, relevant, achievable, and measurable (Hilsden and Verhoef 2004).

There are three main steps to develop your research question. First, you need to *carefully define the problem* you want to address. You may already have significant knowledge about this issue, but specifically defining the problem you want to address greatly increases your chance of actually solving it. This process can also help identify gaps in your understanding of the problem and identify issues you need to consider in your research strategy. Try to start with a specific, narrowly focused problem, which can then be analyzed using a "Cause and Effect" diagram to understand the contributing factors and how they relate to the problem. After defining the problem, you need to *establish you research objectives.* It is helpful to think about the purpose of your research, such as discovering new knowledge, describing phenomena, explaining phenomena, or testing an intervention. From here you can start to consider possible study designs. The third step is to *determine the actual question you want to ask*, and convey it in a clear and concise manner—one sentence if possible. Methodologists have proposed the use of a structured research question. For example, a structured research question about therapy should contain the following five elements: population, intervention, comparator, outcome, and timeframe. These elements are commonly referred to by the acronym PICOT (Haynes 2006). Using the five PICOT elements prompts the investigator to think about the design of the study and the balance between the research question and the feasibility to answer it (Kanji 2015). Keep in mind that you can keep revising your research question as your understanding of the research objectives deepens.

Plan Your Research

After establishing a research question, there are several issues to be addressed as you plan your funding proposal. If you are planning to do a research study, you will need to specify the study design, research protocol, sample size, and data management and statistical analysis plan. Good research projects require high levels of scientific rigor to deliver high quality, believable data. This process takes time and effort, but it will pay great dividends.

Determining what resources you will need for your project is a necessary step when preparing a funding proposal. One of the most important decisions is determining your research team. Based on your research question and objectives, you will need to bring together a team that has the necessary skills and time to devote to your project. Having the right people in the right roles not only maximizes your success, but shows funders that you have the resources and expertise to accomplish your research objectives. The composition of the study team is of particular interest

Table 5.3 Big picture questions to ask before seeking funding

Who are you?	What do you want to do?	How do you want to do it?
• Individual	• Design and develop	• Research
• Affiliate	• Implement	• Collaboration
• Organization	• Build/equip	• Education
• Business	• Scale up	• Innovation

to granting agencies as they must be confident that the project will be completed if they decide to fund it. You will need to include a detailed description of the roles and expertise of each team member in the application. Seeking advisors and mentors early in the process is helpful; their input can save you time and effort. Time is another important resource to consider at this stage; specifically how much time you have to devote to the project, and what additional staff you may need to complete the project. Other important resource considerations include equipment and supplies, access to research space or facilities, and populations in which to test your idea.

All research studies will require an ethical review process such as an Institutional Review Board (IRB). This can take time, often several months, so understanding what is required for your specific research and location is an important step to consider early in the process. Research or projects involving technology innovation have additional considerations such as access to databases, data sharing agreements, and intellectual property issues.

5.1.1.3 Develop Your Funding Strategy

Define the Big Picture

Before starting your search for funding sources, it is important to define the "big picture". Developing clarity about "who you are", "what you want to do", and "how you want to do it", is just as important as developing an achievable and focused research question. Table 5.3 summarizes some of the main categories for each of these questions. Nearly all funders have established parameters regarding the types of organizations and projects they will fund, so understanding your organizational structure and project goals is essential evaluating potential funding opportunities.

Funding Sources

There are several types of funding sources available for research and innovation projects. Grants—"*award of money that allows you to do very specific things that usually meet very specific guidelines that are spelled out in painstaking details and to which you must respond very clearly in your grant proposal*" (Karsh and Fox 2014) are the most commonly sought type of funding source. There are several types of grants: research, innovation, program development, educational and travel. You may want to consider other types of funding sources depending on your answers to the "big picture" questions. Examples include prizes or awards, crowdsourcing and venture capital investor funds, corporate sponsors, and in-kind service and donations. Even if you will not be doing a research study, this framework is still a valuable approach, as most funders will require specific objectives, a clear methodology, and defined outcome measures.

As you start your search, keep in mind that funders usually have very specific requirements for eligibility. The most common categories are specific health conditions or diseases, geographic regions, technologies, and target populations. There are also eligibility requirements related to you and your team such as career stage, previous experience, presence or absence of preliminary data, organization type, and type of project (e.g. research, training, service delivery). Information on potential funders can be found in several different ways. If you are affiliated with a university or other large organization, check to see if you have access to subscription searchable databases of grants or other lists of funding opportunities. Another option is using one of the free databases of grants on the Internet. A good way to start is simply searching directly on the Internet using key words or going directly to the website of a known funder. Many of the best funding opportunities come through personal contacts so "networking" with colleagues and attending conferences can help you find opportunities not available through databases or websites.

Reviewing Funding Announcements

There are many different parameters to review for each potential funding opportunity. First, look at the basic requirements such as the funder's area of interest, application deadlines, geographic restrictions, and applicant eligibility requirements. Once you go through these requirements, the next, and most critical step, is to determine *if the objective of your research or innovation aligns with those of the funder.* In addition to reading the funding announcement very carefully, review the funder's website and previously funded projects to deepen your understanding about their organization and goals. At times, this step can be nuanced, and may require adjusting the emphasis of your research or even reframing your research question or study population to align better with the funder. Even the best written and most compelling application will not be funded if it is does not align with the goals of the funder, so it is wise to think through this step carefully and proceed only if there is a definite match between you and the funder.

Writing a grant application is time consuming, so you want to make sure the funding opportunity meets your needs, too. For example, not all grants will cover salary or travel expenses. If these are necessary for you to proceed, you need confirm that these requirements are eligible. Some grants require matching funds, or require specific collaboration arrangements. It is often possible to contact the funder by email or phone before you start the process in order to fully understand the funder's requirements.

Writing Your Grant

Once you have found a good funding opportunity for your project, you can plan your writing strategy. There are different ways funders request proposals, and are included with the funding announcement, or the "request for proposal" (RFP). This document provides detailed information about eligibility and what the funder is looking to support. It also explains the application process, including deadlines, page limits, and formatting requirements. The content varies widely, but be sure to read and understand everything completely to avoid unnecessary work, or worse yet, having your application rejected due to a technicality. Some funders ask for an initial concept paper. This is a typically a 2, 3 page document with a few questions about your research or project, which the funder uses as a first round screening tool. If they like your idea, you will be invited to submit a full application. You may also be asked to submit a "letter of intent" or LOI, indicating that you plan to submit an application, and is for planning purposes so funders can manage the volume of applications smoothly.

Before you actually start your application, it is a good idea to develop a writing plan so you can complete your application efficiently and on time. Read all the application materials very carefully, creating a list of required documents, and how you will obtain them. It is essential to start early and develop a timeline with due dates, as this endeavor always takes longer than you think. If others will be helping you write the proposal, delegate responsibilities at this early stage. You also need to starting preparing your budget at this early stage. If you have never developed a budget before, it is advisable seek help with this part of the application. If you will be applying through an organization, seek out someone who manages grants as they can help you with planning and writing the budget. In addition, it is also advisable to seek for a person who is familiar with the funding agency platform where the application should be uploaded.

It is very helpful to re-read the application instructions again at this time, and make sure you have a plan to address *all* the specific questions they have requested in the RFP. Your writing style should be clear, succinct, and avoid using jargon or technical terms; quality of content matters more than quantity—excessive length or "wordiness" is not helpful. Perhaps the greatest task the researcher or innovator has, is to "sell" the research idea to potential collaborators, co-investigators, administrators, ethics boards, and ultimately funding agencies. It is important to not only convince them that the project *can* be done, but that it *should* be done and why your study team should be the one to do it. A compelling case can be made by identifying knowledge gaps or the new opportunity your innovation will create using examples, and facts or data.

It is also important to think about how you intend to evaluate and sustain your project. Some important concepts to address include a plan for capturing the lessons learned in the project and how you will share them with the funders, other organizations and the community, a plan for continuing the project after the grant period, and how your project will have a broader impact through replication and scaling up in other locations. Finally, leave plenty of time to revise and edit your content. Ideally, find other investigators or team members to read and critique your application. It can also be helpful to have a reader without direct knowledge of your study area.

5.2 Exercises

5.2.1 Introduction

In this section we describe a series of exercises to guide you through the process of developing your idea into a fundable proposal. Each exercise has worksheets and accompanying documents with more detailed information, templates and checklists (Table 5.4).

5.2.2 Exercise 1: Develop Your Research Question

The research question is the foundation for your entire project. Exercise 1 is a worksheet to guide you through the three main steps to develop your research questions. There are examples of a cause and effect diagram (Ex1.1), a blank template (Ex 1.2), and guidelines on writing a good research question (Ex1.3) (Bordage and Dawson 2003).

Table 5.4 "Toolkit" for developing your funding proposal

Exercise 1	Develop your research question worksheet
	Ex1.1 Cause and effect examples
	Ex1.2 Cause and effect blank template
	Ex1.2 Cause and effect blank template
Exercise 2	Ex2.1 Planning your research
	Ex2.2 Sample timeline
	Ex2.2 Sample timeline
Exercise 3	Funding strategy worksheet
	Ex3.1 Reviewing funding opportunities
	Ex3.2 Finding funding sources
	Ex3.3 Grant writing suggestions

5.2.3 Exercise 2: Research Study Planning Worksheet

Exercise 2 presents the major components of the research study. This includes defining the study population, selecting a research study design, developing a timeline and determining outcome measures. The exercise is accompanied by documents which provide: considerations for planning your research (Ex2.1), a sample timeline (Ex2.2), and an overview of study designs (Ex2.3) (Creswell and Clark 2017). At the completion of the exercise, you should have an initial outline of a fundable grant proposal, and a framework for a research proposal.

5.2.4 Exercise 3: Funding Strategy Worksheet

Exercise 3 is designed to help you develop a funding strategy and search for funding sources. The first part of Exercise 3 guides you through the process of determining what types of funding sources you may want to consider and defining your funding needs for your specific project. The second part of Exercise 3 is a checklist on reviewing funding opportunities, determining if it is a good match, and if your project can meet the requirements of the funding announcement. There are 3 documents to provide additional information: a checklist on reviewing funding announcements (Ex3.1), information regarding finding funding sources including a list of web links to funding sources (Ex3.2), and grant writing suggestions (Ex3.3)

5.3 Uses and Limitations

5.3.1 Various Use Cases

The material in this chapter was originally developed for a workshop for individuals interested in learning more about finding funding for research and technology innovations. It has been revised for use by individuals to develop their own funding proposal, using the worksheets and reference materials provided in the exercises. The original workshop was a half day event with three short presentations introducing the content from the chapter subsections on “The Importance of Research in Mobile Health and Data Science Innovations”, “Developing your mHealth or Data Science Research Project”, and “Develop you Funding Strategy”. The rest of the time was dedicated to working on the exercises in multidisciplinary teams with assistance from the workshop mentors. There is enough content to support a longer event, so participants can present their work to others for feedback and discussion.

5.3.2 Limitations of Information

Getting funding is hard. This chapter will help you be organized and have a clear view on how to succeed in getting your project funded. It provides is an overview of issues that need consideration when planning and funding a research proposal, so it does not cover many of the important details which often determine success or not. The intent is to help researchers and innovators get started, emphasizing the major elements of a successfully funded project. We also recognize that funding sources and opportunities change over time, and that some of the funding links provided may no longer be available.

5.3.3 How this Chapter Links with Other Materials in the Book

In order for any idea or innovation to reach its goal of improved access and quality of health care, it requires significant resources. This chapter aims to provide insight into how researchers and innovators can find and obtain funding so they can transform data science ideas and techniques discussed in the other chapters into usable technologies that can be implemented into the health care delivery system.

References

Bordage, G., & Dawson, B. (2003). Experimental study design and grant writing in eight steps and 28 questions. *Medical Education, 37*(4), 376–385.

Creswell, J. W., & Clark, V. L. P. (2017). *Designing and conducting mixed methods research.* Sage.

Haynes, R. B. (2006). *Clinical epidemiology: How to do clinical practice research* (pp. 3–14). Lippincott Williams & Wilkins. Forming research questions.

Hilsden, R. J., & Verhoef, M. J. (2004). *Writing an effective research proposal.* Retrieved October 4, 2018, from http://people.ucalgary.ca/~rhilsden/Protocol_writing_handout_2004.pdf.

Kanji, S. (2015). Turning your research idea into a proposal worth funding. *The Canadian Journal of Hospital Pharmacy, 68*(6), 458.

Karsh, E., & Fox, A. S. (2014). *The only grant-writing book You'll ever need.* Basic Books a Member of Perseus Books Group.

Kuehn, B. M. (2015). Is there an app to solve app overload? *JAMA, 313*(14), 1405–1407.

Kumar, S., Nilsen, W. J., Abernethy, A., Atienza, A., Patrick, K., Pavel, M., et al. (2013). Mobile health technology evaluation: The mHealth evidence workshop. *American Journal of Preventive Medicine, 45*(2), 228–236.

Labrique, A., Vasudevan, L., Chang, L. W., & Mehl, G. (2013). H_pe for mHealth: more "y" or "o" on the horizon? *International Journal of Medical Informatics, 82*(5), 467–469.

Peters, D. H., Adam, T., Alonge, O., Agyepong, I. A., & Tran, N. (2013). Implementation research: What it is and how to do it. *BMJ, 347,* f6753.

Roess, A. (2017). The promise, growth, and reality of mobile health—Another data-free zone. *New England Journal of Medicine, 377*(21), 2010–2011.

Tomlinson, M., Rotheram-Borus, M. J., Swartz, L., & Tsai, A. C. (2013). Scaling up mHealth: Where is the evidence? *PLoS Medicine, 10*(2), e1001382.

6

System Dynamics Models and CLDs

Gary Lin, Michele Palopoli and Viva Dadwal

Abstract The lack of global data flow in healthcare systems negatively impacts decision-making both locally and globally. This Chapter aims to introduce global health specialists to causal loop diagrams (CLDs) and system dynamics models to help them better frame, examine, and understand complex issues characteristic to data-rich ecosystems. As machine and statistical learning tools become popular among data scientists and researchers, they can help us understand how various data sources and variables interact with each other mechanistically. These complementary approaches go a step beyond machine and statistical learning tools to represent causality between variables affecting data-driven ecosystems and decision-making.

Keywords Data-rich environments · System dynamics · Stock & flow diagrams · Causal loop diagrams · Feedback loops · Statistical learning tools · Data-driven ecosystems

Objectives

This chapter will proceed in three parts. First, in the background, we will describe how system dynamics has suitable applications to data-rich ecosystems. Next, we will share key introductory elements of system dynamics, including CLDs, stock and flow diagrams, and systems modelling. Finally, in the hands-on exercise, we will simulate a system dynamics model of clinical trial data for application in global health.

No prior modelling experience is assumed.

G. Lin
Center for Data Science in Emergency Medicine, School of Medicine, Johns Hopkins University, Baltimore, USA

M. Palopoli
Duke University School of Nursing, Durham, NC, USA

V. Dadwal (✉)
Brooklyn, USA
e-mail: viva.dadwal@gmail.com

6.1 Background

System dynamics is a fundamentally interdisciplinary field of study that helps us understand complex systems and the sources of policy resistance in that system to be able to guide effective change (Sterman 2001). Within system dynamics, causal loop diagrams are the main analytical tools that assist in the identification and visualization of key variables and the connections between them. The related systems modelling methodology of system dynamics involves computer simulation models that are fundamentally unique to each problem setting (Homer and Hirsch 2006: 452).

This section will proceed in three parts. We will introduce, first, what we mean by data-rich ecosystems; second, the terminology of system dynamics; and third, a few applications of system dynamics in data-rich ecosystems.

6.1.1 Data-Rich Ecosystems

Data-rich ecosystems are defined as "technological and social arrangements underpinning the environments in which [data] is generated, analysed, shared and used" (Marjanovic et al. 2017: ii). These systems give rise to dynamic complexity because the system is: (1) constantly changing, (2) tightly coupled, (3) governed by feedback, (4) nonlinear, (5) history-dependent, (6) self-organizing, (7) adaptive, (8) characterized by trade-offs, (9) counterintuitive, and (10) policy resistant (Sterman 2001: 12). Indeed, problems plaguing data-rich ecosystems require understanding how the whole system will react to a seemingly inconsequential modification in one part of the system (Sterman 2001).

One example of such a data-rich ecosystem is global health, where the potential of data holds promise across all the building blocks of health systems. In its broadest sense, health data refers to any type of data that provides use for improved research and innovation, as well as healthcare related decision making (Marjanovic et al. 2017). As a result, a supportive health data ecosystem requires at least the following five elements: (1) collaboration and coordination, (2) public acceptance and engagement with health data, (3) data protection regulation and models of data access and use, (4) data quality, interoperability, and other technical considerations, and (5) workforce capacity (Marjanovic et al. 2017). These complexities, coupled with the still growing landscape of global health data generation, interpretation and use, require a systematic approach that has the potential to facilitate decision-making that aligns our long-term best interests with those of the system as a whole (Sterman 2001).

6.1.2 System Dynamics

A system can be characterized as a group of multiple components that interact with each other. System dynamics was originally meant to invoke systems thinking by endogenizing relevant variables and mathematically connecting causally linked variables (Richardson 2011). In particular, it requires moving away from isolated events and causes and toward the organization of the system as a set of interacting parts (Kirkwood 1998). As a result of its conceptual intuition, the system dynamics paradigm originally came to be interdisciplinary in nature (Sterman 2001). This has notably allowed researchers without quantitative backgrounds to participate in structural formation of the model.

Today, a system dynamics model consists of an interlocking set of differential and algebraic equations developed from a broad spectrum of relevant measured and experiential data (Cavana and Mares 2004). Systems thinking and causal loop diagramming allows researchers to move from conceptual understanding of unidimensional problems to a completed systems model containing scores of such equations, each with their appropriate numerical inputs. Once computerized, these models offer ways of systematically testing policies and scenarios in ways that answer both "what if" and "why" (Homer and Hirsch 2006).

Further, since modelling is iterative, the process relies on repeated attempts of scope selection, hypothesis generation, realistic causal diagramming, quantification, reliability testing, and policy analysis. These steps are selectively repeated until the model is able to generate useful insights while meeting certain requirements, such as its realism, robustness, and flexibility (Homer and Hirsch 2006). Ultimately, the ability to see systems "as a whole" provides a framework for understanding complexity and change, testing levers for policies that would result in sustainable progress (Cavana and Mares 2004; Homer and Hirsch 2006; Senge 1990).

6.1.3 Applications of System Dynamics in Data-Rich Ecosystems

An early application of system dynamics modelling includes an integrated assessment of anthropogenic impacts on the environment and resource scarcity which paved the way for integrated assessment modelling in sustainability applications (Forrester 1961; Meadows et al. 1972). System dynamics models have since found application in a number of data-rich ecosystems. For example, management and business operations benefit from modelling their entire enterprise at a systems-level, which includes all relevant processes, stakeholders, and components. In the context of healthcare delivery, system dynamics have been deployed to address problems with capacity and management of patient flow, but it is not out of the realm of possibilities for system dynamics to be employed as a way to study multiple, mutually reinforcing, interacting diseases and risks, in a way that gives a more realistic snapshot of overall epidemiology and policy implications (Homer and Hirsch 2006). Other successful interventions using system dynamics include long-range market forecasting, strategy development in manufacturing and commercial product development, and models for effective management of large-scale software projects (Sterman 2001).

6.2 Causal Loop Diagrams, Stock and Flow Diagrams, and System Dynamics

This section will give a more thorough introduction to the terminologies, concepts, equations, and tools utilized in system dynamics. The first part will discuss CLDs and, with the use of a classic example, their role in visualizing the relationships that govern complex systems. Then, we will introduce and describe how stock and flow diagrams quantitatively build upon the qualitative relationships mapped out in CLDs. Finally, we briefly discuss the software utilized to simulate and test multiple scenarios for a given system dynamics model.

6.2.1 Causal Loop Diagrams

Social issues that affect people and society typically involve *complex systems* composed of several components and interactions. Thus, answering policy questions typically involves a team of interdisciplinary researchers that observe and discuss the drivers surrounding a certain social issue. In these complex systems, "cause and effect are often distant in time and space, and the delayed and distant consequences of actions are different from and less salient than their proximate effects—or are simply unknown" (Sterman 2001: 16). These components and interactions can be visually mapped using a methodological paradigm or a "language" for understanding the dynamic, interconnected nature of our world, known as CLDs.

CLDs allow researchers to use a systems approach to understand the different scale and scope of an issue. One of the more immediate advantages of CLDs is the intuitive methodology behind building these maps. Indeed, the development of such diagrams or maps (that aim to capture the complexities of a multifaceted issue) do not require extensive quantitative training in engineering or mathematics. Detailed methods for developing CLDs have been outlined by Roberts et al. (1983), Richardson and Pugh (1981), Richardson (1991), Coyle (1996), Sterman (2001), and Maani and Cavana (2004).

For our purposes, the mapping legend to make CLDs comprises two basic features. First, CLDs are composed of variables and directional links (i.e., arrows) that represent causal interactions. The directional links illustrate a "cause and effect" relationship such that the origin variable will affect another variable (i.e., cause → effect).

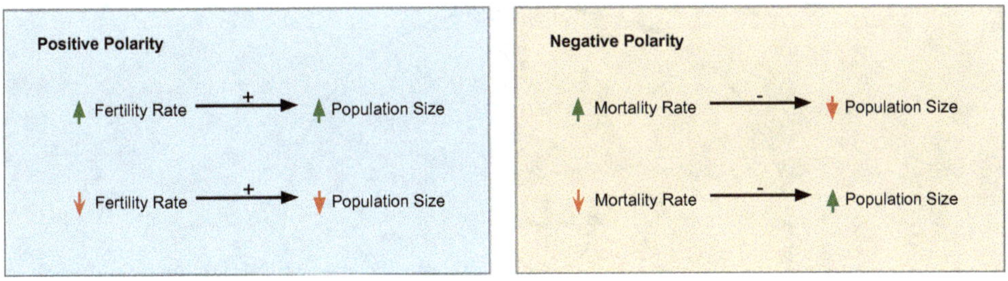

Fig. 6.1 Positive versus negative polarities

Second, causal linkages have two polarities: **positive** (same direction) and **negative** (opposite direction) (Cavana and Mares 2004; Kim 1992; Maani and Cavana 2004; Richardson 1991). A positive causal link indicates that two linked variables will increase or decrease together (same direction). A negative polarity between two variables implies an inverse or opposing relationship (opposite direction); an increase in one variable causes a decrease in the other linked variable and vice versa. In this way, a CLD is developed based on linking variables that are causally related. The following figure represents a simple example that is commonly observed in population modelling (Fig. 6.1).

Once the problem is defined, the next step is to identify the relevant variables that affect the issue. Subsequently, the goal is to identify the variables in the adjacent systems that affect the 'primary variables'. From a graphical standpoint, one can view all the variables in a CLD as 'nodes', and links as 'edges'. After all the variables (nodes) and links are mapped, the 'feedback loops'—or closed loops of variables—become more apparent. A coherent and holistic narrative about a particular problem is created by connecting the nodes and links of several loops (Kim 1992).

Feedback loops are next classified into two categories: **reinforcing** and **balancing**. In literature, reinforcing and balancing feedback loops are sometimes called **positive** and **negative** feedback loops, respectively (Kirkwood 1998). The reinforcing feedback loop is composed of all positive polarities in the same direction and/or an even number of negative polarities in the opposite direction (Kim 1992). If a reinforcing loop has a positive polarity, an even number of negative polarities would simply result in an overall positive polarity (i.e., two sequential links with negative polarity). We demonstrate an example of a reinforcing feedback loop in Fig. 6.2. In this example, we show how a raise in income leads to a rise in savings, in turn, boosting amount of interest accrual. The idea of reinforcing loops is quite provocative since these systems lack nontrivial equilibrium, rendering them unstable.

In contrast, balancing feedback loops exist when a series of variables that are connected in a loop has an odd number of negative polarities. An example of a balancing feedback loop is shown in Fig. 6.3, where we recreated a CLD of the Lotka-Volterra system, which is more commonly known as the 'predator-prey' model. In our example, we show that sheep are prey population and the wolves are the predator population. If there are more wolves, then the population of sheep will decline because the wolves would be consuming more sheep. When there are not enough sheep to

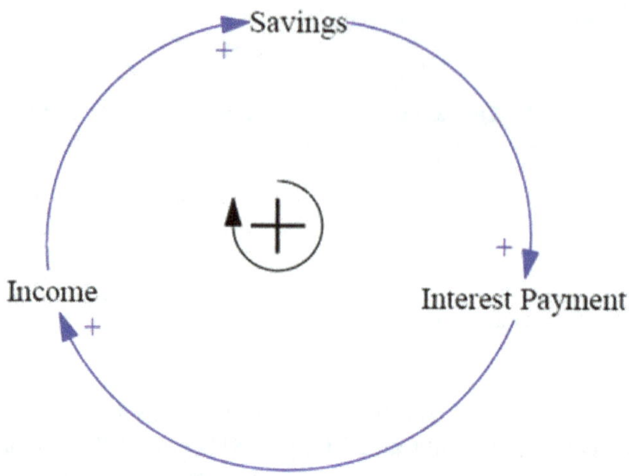

Fig. 6.2 Example of a reinforcing feedback loop (Income and interest on a bank account)

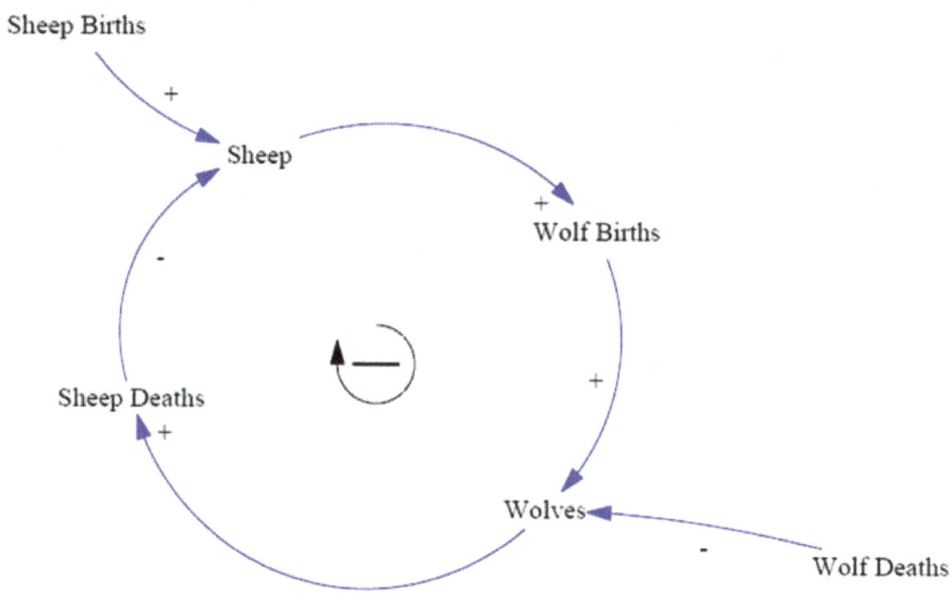

Fig. 6.3 Example of a Lotka-Volterra system of a balancing feedback loop

sustain the consumption requirement of wolves, the wolf population will dwindle. Therefore, this system is inherently a balancing feedback loop because of the inverse relationship between the population of wolves and sheep (Fig. 6.3).

The CLD is constantly analysed visually to identify the key variables and the range of balancing and reinforcing loops it contains. A key feature of this process is also to simplify the conceptual diagram so the resulting insights can be used as the basis for developing and implementing policy (Cavana and Mares 2004). Based on the definition of feedback loops researchers should be able to understand certain mechanisms of a system they are studying. Further, in order for there to be a system that is *stable*, in other words, self-correcting or equilibrium-seeking, there must be a balancing loop that exists in some combination with a reinforcing loop. We encounter many examples of stable systems on a daily basis. For instance, a swinging pendulum eventually returns back to its original resting position (stable equilibrium point) due to gravity and remains stationary after some time.

We can also characterize a system as being *unstable* when a certain variable or mechanism is perturbed from its equilibrium. When a loop loses stability or balancing variables, one must correct the system by adding more counteracting forces. The variables responsible for this instability are typically targets for **policy interventions**. An example of an unstable system includes social dynamics in a country with conflicting groups. In this situation, the equilibrium would be peace. However, peace would be relatively fragile if those groups did not get along with each other. A slight provocation would cause the system to stray away from peace (unstable equilibrium point).

6.2.2 Stock and Flow Diagrams and System Dynamics Modelling

Systems academics have long noted human limitations when dealing with dynamic, evolving, and interconnected systems (Sterman 2001). Stock and flow diagrams and system dynamics modelling can help us avoid mental models that are "static, narrow, and reductionist" (Sterman 2001: 11). Specifically, *dynamic* systems change over time, which necessitates considering the behavior of each variable in a *temporal* domain. This involves translating the visual mapping of CLDs to diagrams that measure the accumulation and dispersal of resources over time (Sterman 2001).

In a stock and flow diagram, there are four main variables: **stock, flow, auxiliary,** and **delay.** A stock variable can be thought of as a "memory" variable which carries over after each time step. Due to their characteristics as defining the "state" of the system, these variables send out signals to all the other parts of the system. For example, one can imagine the volume of water in a container to be a stock variable since the volume in a previous time will carry over into the present unless there is a change in volume, i.e., someone adding more water or draining the container. In contrast, the idea of a changing stock variable can be represented by flow variables. These variables are subject to disappearing if time is hypothetically stopped. Thus, in a situation where the volume of water is increasing due to more water pouring into a container, we can consider that volumetric flow rate as an **inflow** variable. While the volumetric flow loss due to a drainage of the container will be an **outflow** variable. Thus, in Fig. 6.4, stock variables are sheep and wolves, whereas flow variables are Wolf Births, Wolf Deaths, Sheep Births, and Sheep Deaths.

Outside of stock and flow variables, there exist **auxiliary** variables which are simply defined as variables that influence the flows. These variables do not change

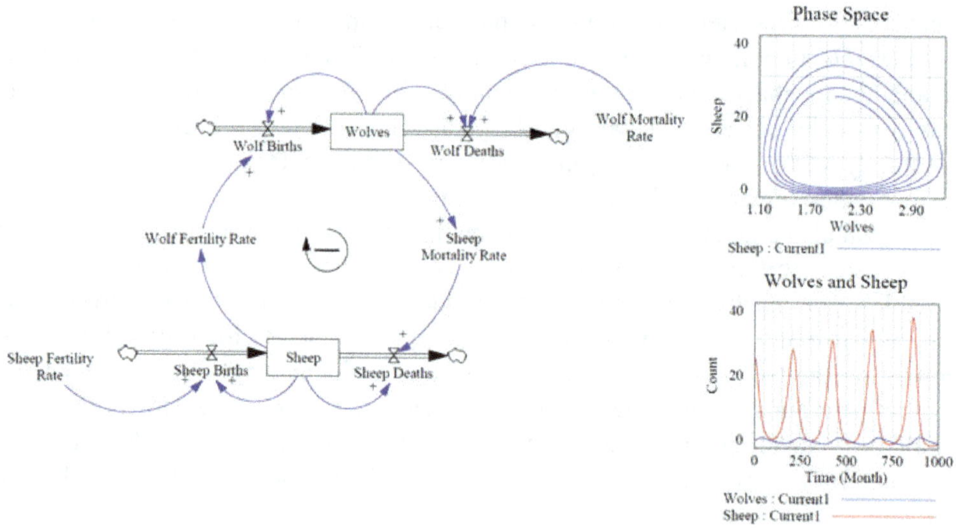

Fig. 6.4 Stock & flow diagram of the Lotka-Volterra model. Assuming arbitrary initial values and constants, the theoretical results of the Lotka-Volterra system were generated using the software Vensim to demonstrate that the stock and flow diagrams is identical to the mathematical formulations. The top right represents the phase space between wolf and sheep populations. The bottom right diagram represent the time series of wolf and sheep populations

the mathematical structure of the system, but do help bring transparency to the model. In the diagram below, auxiliary variables (endogenous) include Wolf Fertility Rate and Sheep Mortality Rate. We also have **constant** values (exogenous) which includes Sheep Fertility Rate and Wolf Mortality Rate.

Lastly, delay variables exist when a casual action occurs at a later time. Delay variables exist when there is a time lag between policy interventions and change in a pattern of human behavior. For example, a tax imposed on a specific good may not result in an immediate decline in demand because it takes time for the consumers to realize and respond to the surge in the price of the good. It should be noted that the delay length itself is a constant that needs to be parameterized and may introduce additional mathematical complexity.

System dynamics models use stock and flow diagrams to translate conceptual models to a mathematical one. Stocks can mathematically be expressed as integrals and generally considered the state variables of the system. Stock variable y can be explicitly represented as:

$$\frac{dy(t)}{dt} = x_{IN}(t) - x_{OUT}(t)$$

$$y(t) = y(t_0) + \int_{t_0}^{t} x_{IN}(\tau) - x_{OUT}(\tau)d\tau \tag{6.1}$$

In Eq. (6.1), the variable x_{IN} is the inflow, and x_{OUT} is the outflow of the system. The combined effect of the inflow and outflow variables represent the derivative of the stock such that inflows are a positive change and outflows are negative change. There could be multiple inflow and outflow variables associated with a stock. As a result, we are able to mathematically solve a system dynamics model as a system of ordinary differential equations. The phase plot and time series plot in Fig. 6.4 were generated using a system dynamics approach with chosen parameters. This was executed by converting stocks and flow diagram of the Lotka-Volterra model into corresponding mathematical equations. The auxiliary variables that determine the inflow of wolves and outflow of sheep are

$$Wolf\ Fertility\ Rate = \alpha \cdot Sheep$$
$$Sheep\ Mortality\ Rate = \omega \cdot Wolves$$

where α and ω are constants.

In stock and flow diagram in Fig. 6.4, the two stocks (represented as the bottom right plots)—Wolves and Sheep—are modified by births and deaths which correspond with the inflow and outflow variables for both stocks and they are described as the following differential equations.

$$\frac{dWolves(t)}{dt} = Wolf\ Births - Wolf\ Deaths$$
$$= Wolf\ Fertility\ Rate \cdot Wolves - Wolf\ Mortality\ Rate \cdot Wolves$$
$$= \alpha \cdot Sheep \cdot Wolves - Wolf\ Mortality\ Rate \cdot Wolves$$

$$\frac{dSheep(t)}{dt} = Sheep\ Births - Sheep\ Deaths$$
$$= Sheep\ Fertility\ Rate \cdot Sheep - Sheep\ Mortality\ Rate \cdot Sheep$$
$$= Sheep\ Fertility\ Rate \cdot Sheep - \omega \cdot Wolves$$

In this predator-prey model, Wolf Mortality Rate and Sheep Fertility Rate will also be considered constants.

6.2.3 Software and Computational Implementation

System dynamics modelling is originally meant to simulate the emerging mechanics and explain a system. Simulation of the mathematical model following the above system conceptualization stages can be undertaken using computers and software. Modern system dynamics modelling software makes it possible for almost anyone to participate in the modelling process. These simulations allow researchers to experiment, test their decision-making skills, and just '*play*' (Sterman 2001: 21).

System dynamics models can be easily implemented in a number of open-source and commercial software such as: Vensim (Free personal learning edition); STELLA (Proprietary); AnyLogic (Proprietary); and NetLogo (Free).

When choosing a suitable software, researchers working in data-rich ecosystems should pay particular attention to the capacity of the program to handle large datasets and advanced analytical tools. R and Python are a favorite for data scientists and researchers because both computing environments are open-source and adept to handling large data (Ihaka and Gentleman 1996; Johansson et al. 2012; McKinney 2013; Pedregosa et al. 2011). Furthermore, these computing languages have access to a wide range of libraries that allow for easy implementation of structural equations modelling.

Although machine learning and probabilistic methods typically perform better in prediction due to their enhanced capabilities of detecting trends in big data, system dynamics models provide more inferential capabilities by allowing researchers to test an expertise-based hypothesis with a complex causal structure. Nevertheless, recent advances in dynamical systems theory has allowed careful and effective parameterization using statistical learning and probabilistic methods (Brunton et al. 2016). Therefore, system dynamics can be robust and incorporate the human domain knowledge and advanced statistical tools. Parameters and initial conditions of the model are usually estimated using statistical means, market research data, analogous product histories, expert opinion, and any other relevant sources of data, quantitative or judgmental (Sterman 2001).

Finally, it is worth mentioning that simulation experiments can suggest the collection of new data and new types of experiments to run to resolve uncertainties and improve the model structure (Sterman 2001). Building model confidence is truly an iterative process that requires robust statistical testing.

6.3 Exercise

Having completed an overview of CLDs, stock and flow diagrams, and system dynamics, this section will now proceed to simulate a system dynamics model for application in global health. Specifically, we apply the system dynamics model to undertake a case study on research data generated by clinical trials, electronic medical records (EMR), and patients. This is an important area of research because movement of data in the global health research system has the potential to impact treatment development globally.

The current premise in global health research is that using clinical trials—and thus using the underlying data for clinical trials—will lead to better treatment development and public health outcomes (Rosala-Hallas et al. 2018). However, in order to bring the right treatment to the right patient at the right time, the process must utilize data from, and contribute data to, a larger global health data ecosystem. Generating real time, pragmatic evidence is not enough; a human-centered data ecosystem will learn from the experience of real patients in real-time, employing all tiers of biological and non-biological data, across therapeutic areas and stakeholders, to better respond to individual and population-based health needs.

Our question seeks to address the relationship between patient EMR data and clinical trial data, and whether the prior can complement existing global health research data sources to enhance our understanding of human disease progression, with the ultimate goal of improving general health outcomes globally. This problem helps us think about the types of policy-based changes that might be necessary for governments, research organizations, and health-service organizations (e.g., providers, hospitals, and clinics) to encourage sharing and use of proprietary data (EMR and clinical trial data). This, we hope, will help identify the types of feedback loops necessary to facilitate better data flows in global health research and make medical breakthroughs benefitting the entire world.

This exercise will proceed in five parts. First, we will identify the key variables in the system. Next, using CLDs and their components (feedback, stock/flow, time delay, non-linearity), we conceptually visualise the ways in which data flows within the current global health research system are conceived. Equations were logically derived using variables and developed CLDs. These equations were next computationally modeled using R. Lastly, we share the types of policy questions and directions that may be run on the model.

6.3.1 Identifying the System and Variables

When choosing variables, it is important to use variables that describe patterns of behaviour and activity in global health, rather than specific singular events (Kim 1992). Further, it can be helpful to think about the types of variables that affect the problem the most, and which the least. In this regard, subject matter experts should be consulted to broadly identify key factors affecting the model in the form of expert elicitation.

In our case study, four stock variables were ultimately decided as being critical to the movement of data within the global health landscape. Specifically, patients in hospitals, shared EMR data, health research data, and available treatments were all identified as key recurring variables contributing to the data-rich ecosystem of global health. These four variables were chosen because we are interested in the amount of data generated (EMR and clinical) and the impact data has on public health and research (patients and treatment availability). Further, these variables represent the units of measure for data (Shared EMR data and Health Research Data), as well as a surrogate measure for general health (Patients in hospitals) and scope of health products (Available treatments).

Efforts were taken to brainstorm some of the key factors that would affect the aforementioned stock variables (Table 6.1). In a real exercise, these factors would be consulted upon by experts to confirm their suitability for the model, including whether they could be easily measured and monitored. Moreover, it must be mentioned that

Table 6.1 Brainstorming variables for systems conceptualization

	Factors causing growth	Factors causing decline
Shared EMR data	Technologies (devices) that measure RT data; interoperability of devices and health systems (data from patient wearables automatically uploaded to record); more patients in hospitals; early EMR capture (time-based input, birth-to-death); paid data (individuals could sell their own data)	Negative patient perspectives (privacy and mistrust); time taken to collect data; poor infrastructure (devices and hospital systems not lined up/interoperable)
Health research data	Number of clinical trials; low cost of clinical trials; less regulatory barriers to conducting CT; cooperation between research companies; inclusion of different types of data (failure data); funder requirement for data sharing; computer and animal modelling	Exclusivity clauses between pharma companies; IP rights; less clinical trials (due to high cost, over-regulation, poor trial enrollment, poorly designed trials; IRB approval); cyber attacks; funder restrictions on data sharing
Patients in hospitals	Sick people; hospital mergers and acquisitions; referrals; improved patient perceptions (high quality care, and overcoming historical fears); population demographics (old age, low socioeconomic status, or poor quality food); diseases and epidemics; environment; public health/epidemiology failure; bad vaccination predictions/crops and patient perceptions of vaccines	Prevention, better primary care, population demographics (characteristics associated with better worse outcomes); personalized care; no insurance
Available treatments	Clinical trial success; approval rate; encouraging innovation environment; number of clinical trials (lower cost of research, governmental incentives, funding, trained research workforce, clinical trial design); regulatory environment	Adverse events/toxicity; recall based on post-market surveillance; less clinical trials (cost of research, no funding/incentives, lack of workforce, poorly designed clinical trials); legal and regulatory barriers (ethical/moral constraints); cost of drugs; manufacturing issues (ingredient shortage, and GMP violations)

a number of variables were decidedly not included in the system conceptualization of global health research, including disease prevention, intellectual property governance, research infrastructure, and workforce.

6.3.2 *Causal Loop Diagrams (Feedback, Stock/Flow, Time Delay, Non-linearity)*

Next, we proceed to establishing the links between the stock variables on the CLD, the polarity or direction on each link, stocks and flows, and the identification and labelling of the reinforcing or balancing loops in the diagram. For example, we know that one of the primary causal links that drives public health outcomes is the number of *approved treatments* (stock variable) with an inflow variable called *approval rate.* Similarly, approval rates are affected by research productivity and total number of clinical trials—both reinforcing loops. On the other hand, research and development budgets have a balancing effect on the total available treatments.

We have identified two balancing loops in Fig. 6.5. These are loop B1, indicated by the red counter-clockwise arrow, and loop B2 indicated by the clockwise arrow (Fig. 6.5). B1 regulates the amount of EMR data being generated, and B2 helps control the amount of patients that gets admitted into the hospital. The reinforcing loop R1 is seen as amplifying the system, which through the positive (+) signs at the arrowheads indicate that the effect is reinforcing in a positive direction. We only show these three feedback loops to demonstrate examples but it is worth noting that this CLD contains other feedback loops that also contribute to the behavior of the system.

In our hypothetical system, we assumed the hospital directly collect the data from the patients and their EMR. The patients have the right to share their data which

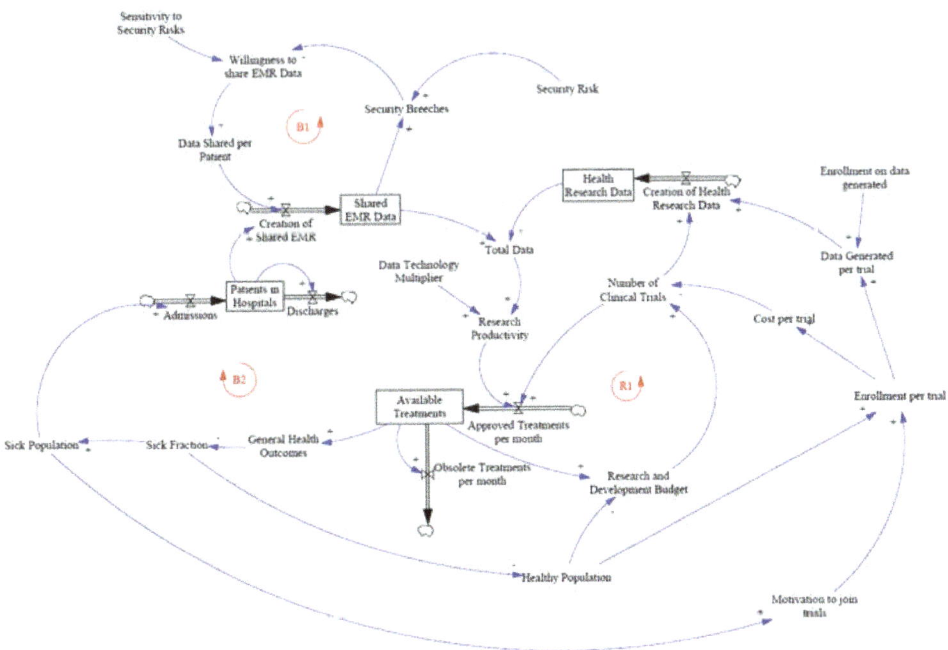

Fig. 6.5 CLD showing data flow in global health research

determines the amount of data that should be shared; however, the amount of data that is shared is influenced by their *willingness* to share their own data. As an example, the threat of cyber attacks on EMR systems impact the patients' willingness to share. This effect is captured by the feedback loop B1. In loop B2, the single negative polarity between general health outcomes and sick fraction causes the entire feedback loop to be a balancing. This loop signifies the tradeoff between number of sick people in hospitals generating data that contributes to treatment development and general health outcomes. In other words, it is assumed that having a healthy-only population would stall the treatment development process.

In feedback loop R1, we assume that pharmaceutical companies are the sole sponsors of clinical trials, having direct access to both EMR and clinical trial data (health research data). The number of available treatments is directly linked to research & development budget. Furthermore, we assumed that *all* of the research & development budget is spent on conducting clinical trials (represented as number of clinical trials) in each time period. The cost of clinical trials is positively correlated with number of enrolled subjects in clinical trials (enrollment per trial).

Although a host of other variables and loops, both reinforcing and balancing, could be identified as being relevant in the process, care was given to keep the conceptual diagram as simple as possible in order to ensure a parsimonious model. Thus, only the dominant loops were reflected in the CLD, which signify the behaviour of the system shifting from acceleration to deceleration, and gradual equilibrium. As mentioned, the CLD may be revised and a number of times as understanding deepens and the multidisciplinary process unfolds.

6.3.3 Constructing System Dynamics Equations

Based on the CLD/stock & flow diagram that we developed in Fig. 6.5, we can formulate the conceptual model into mathematical equations. To illustrate how one would formulate a stock and flow equation, let us look at the stock variable '*patients in hospitals*'.

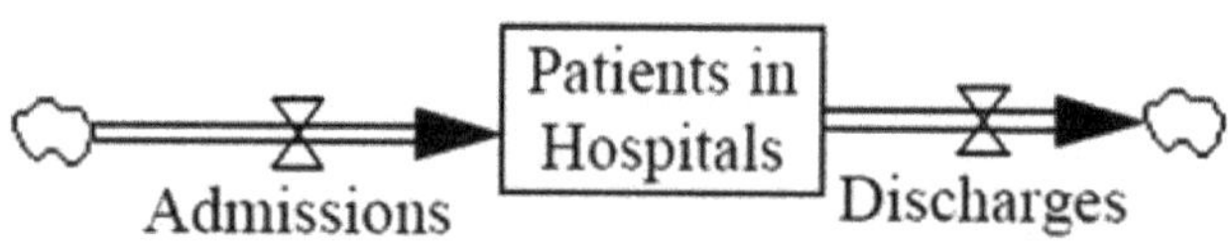

For *patients in hospitals* P, we can deduce that there are primarily an inflow and outflow: *Admissions* IP and *Discharges* OP. We assume that no one dies in our fictional hospital. As a result, our equation looks like the following:

$$\frac{dP(t)}{dt} = IP(t) - OP(t) \tag{6.2}$$

The inflow, admissions IP, in our model is simply equal to the *sick population* SP (auxiliary variable), which makes the assumption that all sick person go directly to the hospital in our fictional world. For real life applications, we could include a delay variable and/or constraint on the impact of sick people on hospital admissions. Thus,

$$IP(t) = SP(t) \tag{6.3}$$

While the outflow, discharges OP, can be a function of patients if we model it as a fraction, λ, being discharged from the hospital. As mentioned previously, this value is being subtracted in Eq. (6.2) because it is an outflow.

$$OP(t) = \lambda \cdot P(t) \tag{6.4}$$

As a result, we substitute IP and SP and rewrite the differential equation for stock variable, P, as

$$\frac{dP(t)}{dt} = SP(t) - \lambda \cdot P(t) \tag{6.5}$$

It also worth mentioning that if we continue substituting auxiliary variables into the flow variables of our stock differential equations, we can mathematically reduce the entire model into a system of only four differential equations because our system only has four stock variables, and each differential equation corresponds with a stock variable.

We present several examples in the following paragraphs to illustrate the logic behind formulating a balancing feedback loop. This includes three auxiliary variables, one inflow variable, and one stock variable based on expert knowledge. Take a look at the balancing feedback loop B1, highlighted in Fig. 6.6:

Since security risk α is fixed in our model, we assume that if more people share their data that would lead to a frequency of security breaches. Therefore, *security breaches* S is defined as a function of *security risk* (percentage of data that is compromised) and the amount of *shared EMR data* D_S.

$$S(t) = \alpha \cdot D_S(t) \tag{6.6}$$

In turn, security breaches *negatively* affect the *willingness to share EMR data* WS which follows the logic that less people are willing to share their personal information if they observe higher incidences of security threats. This negative polarity enables feedback loop B1 to be balancing. Therefore, we must choose a mathematical function that has an inverse relationship between the dependent and independent variable. As a result, we can express an inverse mathematical relationship between WS and S as

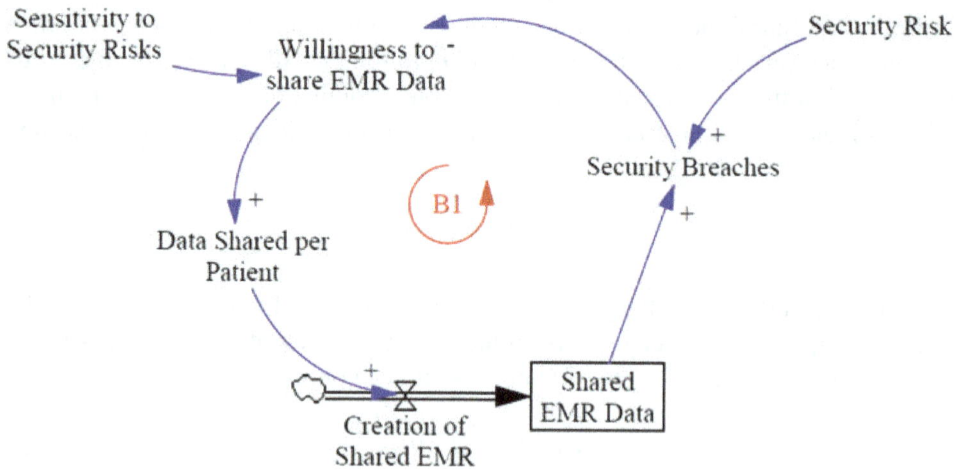

Fig. 6.6 Feedback loop B1

$$WS(t) = \frac{1}{\beta \cdot S(t)} \tag{6.7}$$

where β is the *sensitivity of patients to security risks*. The willingness to share data positively influence the data shared by each patient (labeled as *data shared per patient* and symbolized as $\widehat{D_S}$).

$$\widehat{D_S}(t) = \gamma \cdot WS(t) \tag{6.8}$$

Proceeding along the link, we get to the inflow variable, *creation of shared EMR data* ID_S which is the number of patients P multiplied by the data shared per patient $\widehat{D_S}$

$$ID_S(t) = \widehat{D_S}(t) \cdot P(t) \tag{6.9}$$

Finally, the creation of shared EMR data directly feeds into the shared EMR data stock.

$$\frac{dD_S(t)}{dt} = ID_S(t) \tag{6.10}$$

For a complete listing of all the equations in our model, please refer to the supplement Jupyter notebook.

6.3.4 Modelling and Data Integration

As we have demonstrated, we can convert our CLD/stock and flow diagram into a system dynamics model by prescribing each causal link with a mathematical equation. After populating each link with an equation, we are able to numerically solve the entire of system as a set of ordinary differential equations using previously developed methods to solve differential equations.

The system dynamics model that was described in the previous section was implemented in R, a statistical programming environment. As previously mentioned, R is a robust programming language that allows users to develop their own numerical solver or access a wide variety of libraries that are useful for statistical analysis and numerical methods. In our example, we used the library package **deSolve** (Soetaert et al. 2010) and **FME** (Soetaert and Petzoldt 2010) to, compute the dynamic behavior and parameterize our coefficients, respectively. To solve these models, we would need to employ a numerical method (e.g., forward and backward-stepping Euler's method, or Runge-Kutta family of solvers). These solvers have been programmed in the **deSolve** library in R which makes it easy to implement into any system dynamics model. The reader may refer to the accompanying Jupyter notebook located in the following URL that contains the steps needed to implement the system dynamics model: https://github.com/scarygary89/SimpleHealthDataSharingSD/blob/master/HealthDataSharingModel.ipynb.

System dynamics models can be developed to formalize logic without much data. However, the model's usefulness is greatly enhanced if the parameters can be determined based on a maximum likelihood estimation and finding the confidence intervals using likelihood methods or bootstrapping (Dogan 2007). The parameters that we adjust to fit the model are the constant variables system dynamics model. There may also be times where initial values are also considered a parameter. Figure 6.7 shows how fitted parameters produce a simulated trendline (teal line) compares with "actual data" (red points). For demonstration purposes, the data in Fig. 6.7 is generated synthetically and not based on any real dataset.

The resulting parameter values based on the calibration and fit is located in the following Table 6.2.

Based on these constants, we have enough information to replicate the model and develop a baseline scenario in which we can test alternative policy scenarios. These parameters are estimated based on maximum likelihood estimation that calibrates a parameter that minimizes the (errors) residuals to best fit the data.

Error analysis can be conducted to calculate standard statistical measures that are similar to regression models. We can conduct hypothesis testing on each parameter by assuming a null hypothesis that a parameter is equal to zero and testing that against alternative hypothesis the parameter is equal to the calibrated value and comparing the error distributions—this allows us to conduct a t-test and calculate p-values assuming normality in error distribution. Other parameter validation methods include bootstrapping (refer to Rahmandad et al. 2015a) and method of simulated

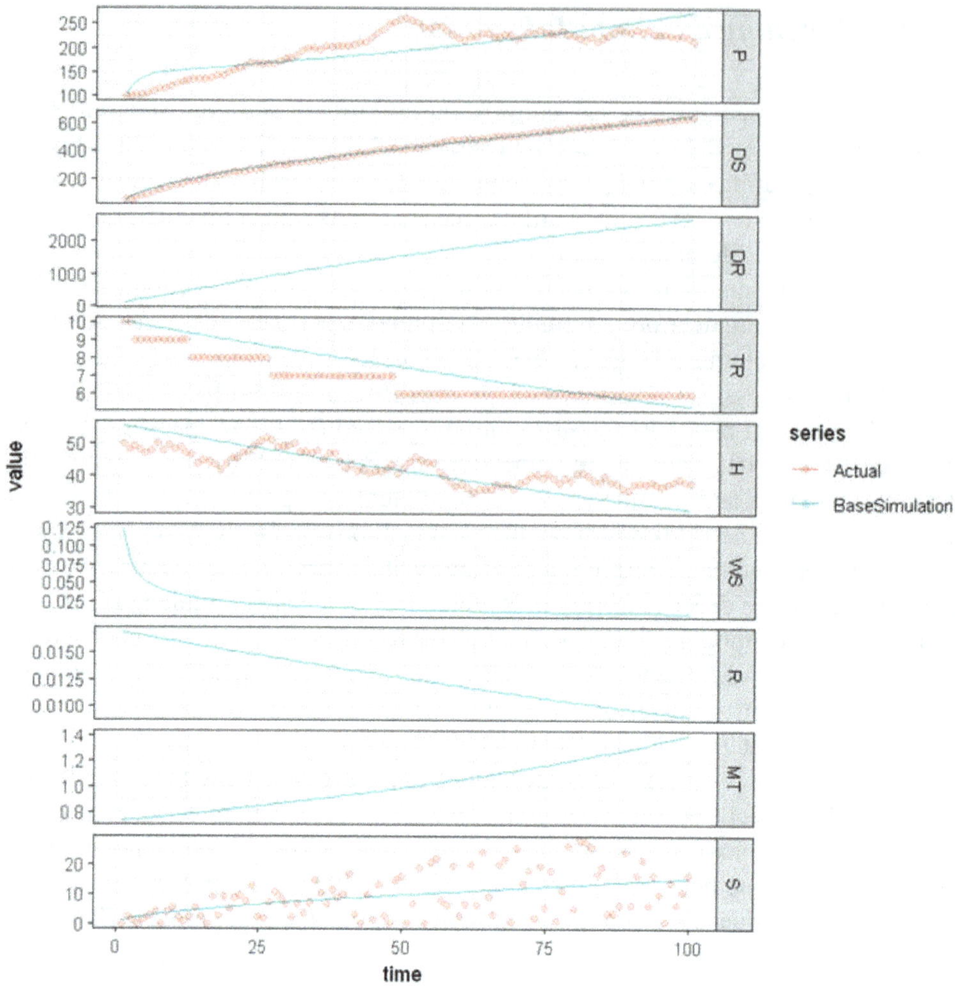

Fig. 6.7 Model results. Dynamic trendlines (teal line) of our system dynamics model for the four stock variables (patients in hospitals P, shared EMR data D_S, health research data D_R, and available treatments TR) and five auxiliary variables (general health outcomes H, willingness to share WS, research & development budget R, motivation to join a clinical trial MT, and security breaches S) compared with data points (red points)

moments (refer to Rahmandad et al. 2015b) which can help the modeler build confidence in the estimation of each parameter. To further understand the parameters and their sensitivities, the modeler may wish to perform a Monte Carlo Markov Chain (MCMC) analysis (refer to Rahmandad et al. 2015c).

6.3.5 *Interpreting Results and Policy Directions*

Once the model is calibrated and running, researchers may wish to use it for testing targeted policy questions. For the purposes of this exercise, we are less concerned

Table 6.2 Parameter values based on model fitting with data

Parameter	Value	Definition
α	0.0234	Security risk (percentage)
β	6.931	Sensitivity to security risks
γ	1.774	Unrestricted data sharing
δ	5.582	Availability of treatment on general health
ζ	12.154	Inverse relationship between general health and sickness frequency
η_1	11.388	Data technology multiplier
ρ	84.78	Market success on R&D budget
ν	0.010	Cost per subject
σ	54.69	Clinical trials multiplier
θ	0.010	Sick population effect on enrollment motivation
λ	0.500	Hospital discharge rate
μ	0.010	Trial enrollment size on data generated per trial
μ	20.477	Obsolete treatment fraction

with the actual results since we are only illustrating the types of questions that may be of interest to global health policy-makers wishing to utilize system dynamics.

Three particular insights produced from our hypothetical CLD led us to consider the impact of cyber security attacks (security risk); data capture and interoperability in clinical trials (data generated per trial), and machine learning and artificial algorithms (data technology) on the global health research system. These areas of interest led us to propose the kinds of questions that may be run on the model we have generated:

- Assuming an increase in data security attacks, where can policy-makers best target resources to ensure patient's continue to contribute health data?
- How might birth-to-death collection of data impact the cost of clinical trials? How does the collection of data both from sick and healthy people impact the price of clinical trials?
- How much money can be invested in new data technology to result in a two-fold decrease of patients in hospitals?

6.4 Uses and Limitations

Our generation faces unimagined levels of information generated every second by new and existing actors. System dynamics complement existing modelling and simulation methodologies to navigate policy questions affecting data-rich ecosystems. Unlike the predictive and explanatory powers of machine learning and probabilistic methods, system dynamics is simply a tool for formalizing and quantifying complex relationships.

Like all models, system dynamics models are 'wrong' due to their inherent inability to understand *all* of the complex relationships and limitations of human rationality. It must be noted that modelling complex systems require an understanding of the dynamic behavior of variables and the range of possible parameter values which can lead to system uncertainties. System dynamics attempts to understand complexity by incorporating knowledge of modeler and its collaborators into a logical formalism that allows for a mathematical structure to be developed. However, parameterization of a complex model can be difficult due to the "curse of dimensionality" and some have propose methods to deal with this issue (Bellman 1957; Ye and Sugihara 2016). Finally, the validation of system dynamics models depends on availability of data and the opinions of domain experts. For more information on this topic, please refer to others who have written comprehensive reviews of the limitations of system dynamics (Featherston and Doolan 2012).

Acknowledgements The authors would especially like to thank Dr. Sauleh Siddiqui for his guidance in the development of this work. The ideas in this chapter were developed as a result of the broader Clinical Trials System Project (CTSP), a multi-year effort led by MIT Collaborative Initiatives in partnership with Johns Hopkins University. The overall CTSP mission is to apply a systems based analysis to the clinical trial system. The project was generously funded through gifts from Bloomberg Philanthropies, Blakely Investment Corporation, the Argosy Foundation, and the Kelly Family Foundation. For more information, please visit clinicaltrials.jhu.edu.

References

Bellman, R. (1957). *Dynamic programming*. Princeton, NJ: University Press.

Brunton, S. L., Proctor, J. L., & Kutz, J. N. (2016). Discovering governing equations from data by sparse identification of nonlinear dynamical systems. *Proceedings of the National Academy of Sciences, 113*(15), 3932–3937. https://doi.org/10.1073/pnas.1517384113.

Cavana, R. Y., & Mares, E. D. (2004). Integrating critical thinking and systems thinking: From premises to causal loops. *System Dynamics Review, 20*(3), 223–235. https://doi.org/10.1002/sdr.294.

Coyle, R. G. (1996). *System dynamics modelling: A practical approach*. New York: Chapman & Hall/CRC.

Dogan, G. (2007). Bootstrapping for confidence interval estimation and hypothesis testing for parameters of system dynamics models. *System Dynamics Review, 23*(4), 415–436. https://doi.org/10.1002/sdr.362.

Featherston, C., & Doolan, M. (2012) A critical review of the criticisms of system dynamics. In *The 30th International Conference of the System Dynamics Society*, St. Gallen, Switzerland, 22 July 2012. Retrieved from https://www.systemdynamics.org/assets/conferences/2012/proceed/papers/P1228.pdf.

Forrester, J. (1961). *Industrial dynamics*. Cambridge, MA: MIT Press.

Homer, J. B., & Hirsch, G. B. (2006). System dynamics modeling for public health: Background and opportunities. *American Journal of Public Health, 96*(3), 452–458. https://doi.org/10.2105/AJPH.2005.062059.

Ihaka, R., & Gentleman, R. (1996). R: A language for data analysis and graphics. *Journal of Computational and Graphical Statistics, 5*(3), 299–314. https://doi.org/10.1080/10618600.1996.10474713.

Johansson, J. R., Nation, P. D., & Nori, F. (2012). QuTiP: An open-source Python framework for the dynamics of open quantum systems. *Computer Physics Communications, 183*(8), 1760–1772. https://doi.org/10.1016/j.cpc.2012.02.021.

Kim, D. H. (1992, February). Guidelines for drawing causal loop diagrams. *The Systems Thinker.* Retrieved November 20, 2018, from https://thesystemsthinker.com/guidelines-for-drawing-causal-loop-diagrams-2/.

Kirkwood, C. W. (1998). System behavior and causal loop diagrams. In: *System dynamics methods: A quick introduction* (pp. 1–14).

Maani, K. E., & Cavana, R. Y. (2004). *Systems thinking and modelling: Understanding change and complexity*. Albany: Pearson Education.

Marjanovic, S., Ghiga, I., Yang, M., et al. (2017). Understanding value in health data ecosystems: A review of current evidence and ways forward. *RAND Corporation.* https://doi.org/10.7249/RR1972.

McKinney, W. (2013). *Python for data analysis*. Beijing: O'Reilly.

Meadows, D. H., Meadows, D. L., Randers, J., et al. (1972). *The limits to growth: A report for the club of rome's project on the predicament of mankind*. New York, NY: Universe Books.

Pedregosa, F., Varoquaux, G,, & Gramfort, A., et al. (2011). Scikit-learn: Machine learning in Python, *12,* 2825–2830.

Rahmandad, H., Oliva R., & Osgood, N. D. (Eds). (2015a). Chapter 1: Parameter estimation through maximum likelihood and bootstrapping methods. In: *Analytical methods for dynamic modelers* (pp. 3–38). MIT Press.

Rahmandad, H., Oliva R., & Osgood, N. D. (Eds). (2015b). Chapter 2: Using the method of simulated moments for system identification. In: *Analytical methods for dynamic modelers* (pp. 39–70). MIT Press.

Rahmandad, H., Oliva R., & Osgood, N. D. (Eds). (2015c). Chapter 5: Combining Markov chain Monte Carlo approaches and dynamic modeling. In: *Analytical methods for dynamic modelers* (pp. 125–169). MIT Press.

Richardson, G. P. (1991). *Feedback thought in social science and systems theory.* Philadelphia: University of Pennsylvania Press.

Richardson, G. P. (2011). Reflections on the foundations of system dynamics. *System Dynamics Review, 27*(3), 219–243. https://doi.org/10.1002/sdr.462.

Richardson, G. P., & Pugh, A. L. (1981). *Introduction to system dynamics modeling with dynamo.*, MIT Press/Wright-Allen series in system dynamics Cambridge, MA: MIT Press.

Roberts, N., Anderson, D. F., Deal, R. M., et al. (1983). *Introduction to computer simulation: The system dynamics approach.* Reading, MA: Addison-Wesley.

Rosala-Hallas, A., Bhangu, A., & Blazeby, J., et al. (2018). Global health trials methodological research agenda: Results from a priority setting exercise. *Trials* 19(1). https://doi.org/10.1186/s13063-018-2440-y.

Senge, P. M. (1990). *The fifth discipline: The art and practice of the learning organization* (1st ed.). New York: Doubleday/Currency.

Soetaert K, P. T., & Setzer, R. W. (2010). *Solving differential equations in R* (Vol. 33, No. 9). Retrieved from https://EconPapers.repec.org/RePEc:jss:jstsof:v:033:i09.

Soetaert, K., & Petzoldt, T. (2010). Inverse modelling, sensitivity and Monte Carlo analysis in *R* using package **FME**. *Journal of Statistical Software, 33*(3), 1–28. https://doi.org/10.18637/jss.v033.i03.

Sterman, J. D. (2001). System dynamics modeling: Tools for learning in a complex world. *California Management Review, 43*(4), 8–25. https://doi.org/10.2307/41166098.

Ye, H., & Sugihara, G. (2016). Information leverage in interconnected ecosystems: Overcoming the curse of dimensionality. *Science, 353*(6302), 922–925. https://doi.org/10.1126/science.aag0863.

7

Digital Health and the Usage of Blockchain

Philip Christian C. Zuniga, Rose Ann C. Zuniga, Marie Jo-anne Mendoza, Ada Angeli Cariaga, Raymond Francis Sarmiento and Alvin B. Marcelo

Abstract We present in this chapter discussion of how blockchain can be used in Digital Health. Benefits and risks of using blockchain were presented. Guide questions with sample answers are also presented to deepen the discussion of the topic. At the last section of the chapter, several use cases on how blockchain is used in Digital Health are presented.

Keywords Blockchain · Crytography · Data security · Data trust

Learning Objectives

(1) Describe how public and private blockchain works
(2) Propose and evaluate blockchain use cases in healthcare

7.1 Introduction

Blockchain technology has been known since the early 1990's through the work of Stuart Haber and W. Scott Stornetta. In their work, *How to Time Stamp a Document* (Haber and Stornetta 1991), the authors propose a methodology to time stamp document using cryptography to prevent counterfeiting of crucial documents. The first real implementation of blockchain was done by Satoshi Nakamoto in 2008 (Nakamoto 2008). His work was focused on using blockchain in cryptocurrencies.

Blockchain revolves on the idea of having a decentralized system of storing data, where each participant/node will have a copy of the ledger of transactions done. By doing so, it will be impossible for someone to alter data in the blockchain without informing other participants. This also eliminates the need for a centralized system that handles all the data since all participants would have their own copies (Zheng et al. 2017). Usually, blockchain is very useful in scenarios where there is a strong centralized entity. In this work, we discuss how blockchain can be used in Digital Health.

P. C. C. Zuniga (✉) · R. A. C. Zuniga · M. J. Mendoza · A. A. Cariaga · R. F. Sarmiento · A. B. Marcelo
Standards and Interoperability Lab-Asia, Mandaluyong City, Philippines
e-mail: phil@sil-asia.org

Blockchain is expected to change the way how Digital Health is done. Digital health implementations rely heavily on centralized systems. This can be seen in the need to validate data, in having a regulatory body and in securing patient data. All of these can be transformed by blockchain. In a survey made by the *European Coordination Committee of the Radiological, Electromechanical and Healthcare IT industry*, several areas are identified to be a good pilot use case for blockchain (COCIR 2017).

(1) Supply Chains
(2) Drug Verification
(3) Claims Reimbursement
(4) Access Control
(5) Clinical Trials

In this workshop, we will present a framework on evaluating blockchain use cases and examine whether the above-mentioned use cases would also be able to pass the evaluation parameter. We will also present a sample use case for a personal health record system using blockchain.

7.2 A Discussion on Blockchain

There are two main important ideas in blockchain.

1. Blockchain consists of a list of blocks that are cryptographically linked with one another.
2. All participant nodes in the system have a copy of the blockchain.

Each blockchain block generally consists of three main parts: [1] the transaction data, [2] the hash of the previous block and [3] the hash of the current block. Each block is connected since every block contains the hash of the previous block hence would have a way to access the previous block. Instead of storing the blockchain in a single centralized node, copies of the blockchain are distributed to each participant nodes. Participants can add a block, and this block will also be added to the copies of other participants.

Because of these properties, blockchain is immutable. Any modification done on the blockchain will change the hash values of the succeeding blocks, and all the changes in the hash values should be reflected in the copies of the participants. The immutability of the blocks in blockchain ensures that the data saved are authentic as stored by the participant. However, this does not ensure that the correct participants will send the correct data. Blockchain works on this issue either by making other participants validate the data submitted by one participant or by only allowing authorized participants to store data in it.

Blockchain can be categorized as *public* or *private* blockchain. For public blockchains, anyone can send data to the blockchain, but this data will need to be validated by other participants. Private blockchain on the other hand is a limited form of blockchain as only a select member can send data to the blockchain. Another category for blockchains, which is also similar to the earlier classification are permissioned and permissionless blockchain. Permissioned blockchain requires certain permissions before a participant submits a data on blockchain. A permissionless blockchain on the otherhand allows participants to add data to the blockchain without the necessary permissions. In usual blockchain models, public blockchains work with permissioned models, since everyone can add data to the blockchain, and thus permissions must first be checked if the data can be added. On the otherhand, private blockchains usually work with permissionless blockchains, since there is an assumption that users in private blockchains are already authenticated and authorized, hence no additional validation step is done.

Guide Questions:

(1) What benefits of blockchain can be used to leverage against Centralized Systems?
(2) Are there any trade offs in using blockchain?
(3) What are the advantages/disadvantages of permissionless/permissioned or public/private blockchain?

Suggested Answers:

(1) Three benefits can be identified when using blockchain as compared to Centralized systems. Blockchain does not require back-ups since every participant have a copy of the chain. It is not a single point of failure component, and there is no single source of truth.
(2) The main trade off in using blockchain is the computational overhead due to the need to synchronize data with other participants. If validation of data is needed (i.e. Proof work/Proof of stake) then it will add significant computational overhead too.
(3) There is less computational overhead when using permissioned or private blockchains since the validation stage can be removed. There are also less participants since these participants would require authentication/permission credentials. Public/permissionless blockchain allows everyone to push data to the chain. This is more open; however, validation of data will still be required.

7.3 When to Use Blockchain?

Blockchain is a solution that can solve many issues in data management and data storage. However, it is not a solution to every problem. There are overheads to using blockchain, and it is important that its used is maximized to make it a viable alternative to existing systems. In this section, we will present some properties of a use case that will benefit greatly from blockchain.

1. Data sharing is required. A blockchain based approach is viable if the use case requires participants to share data to other entities. Data sharing allows the content of the data to be validated and authenticated by other users. Since data is immutable in blockchain, it will be easier for the receiving entity to validate the data since there is a presumption that this data was not altered illegally.
2. Multiple parties modifying a single database. Another use case property that benefits from blockchain is when multiple parties need to modify a single database. Since modifications done in blockchain are broadcasted to all participants, the data provenance is kept and recorded.
3. Trust on the data. Given that data is shared and multiple parties modify the data, it is important that participants can still trust it. Without blockchain, it will be not inherent for the data integrity to be maintained, and additional steps are needed to ensure the integrity. In blockchain, given that there are ways to validate the data or authenticate the participants first, data stored in the blockchain can always be assumed as true. Also unlike existing systems where a centralized database becomes the single source of truth, in blockchain, any copy of the chain that is with any of the participants can be a trustworthy source of truth.
4. Security is of utmost importance. Use cases where security is important benefits greatly in blockchain since data may be encrypted (data privacy), it may not be modified without informing other participants (data integrity), and participants need either to prove validity of data (authentication) or would need to have the proper credentials before submitting data (authorization).

Guide Questions:

(1) Will a general healthcare workflow of sharing of patient data benefit from blockchain?

Suggested Answer:

Usually, healthcare workflows require multiple parties accessing and modifying patient data. This may include: doctors, pharmacists, nurses, lab technicians, and even insurance providers. Patient data can also be shared to multiple entities either as individual data (i.e. insurance) or aggregated with the population (i.e. disease surveillance). Also, validity/correctness of the data is important as practitioners should believe that data written by other doctors on the patient's well being is correct. Or insurance agencies must be able to confirm that the medical abstract provided by doctors truly reflect the status of the patient.

It is also important to note that health data is currently the most prized data by hackers. Recent studies have valued the cost of a single health record to up to 400 USD, [5] and this is higher than the per record cost of financial or commercial data. This implies the need of securing health data.

Given how current health care information systems work, and given the trend where patient data is shared across different stakeholders, it follows that blockchain is really something that can improve how health information systems, particularly health information exchanges, work.

7.4 Challenges in Using Blockchain

Despite the benefits obtained in using blockchain, there are still many identified challenges, both technically and legally, in using blockchain. The following are the primary challenges:

1. Scalability Issues

Since increase in the number of participants lead to increase in the number of transactions, scalability has been one of the leading issues in the use of blockchain. It is projected that there is an exponential growth in the number of transactions in Bitcoin. The scalability issue in blockchain stems from the fact that each participant receives a copy of the blockchain hence an increase in the number of participants increases the number of transactions and the number of blockchain copies that need to be updated every time a new transaction is made.

2. Data Migration

Using blockchain is premised to an assumption that the data that will be used are already in digital format. Migrating from a system that is totally manual is a lot harder when the migration is towards a blockchain based solution as data will need to be structured such that it can be processed by blockchain.

3. Registration of New Participants

Another premise in blockchain use is that all participants in blockchain must have a copy of the chain. This will create additional complexity when participants (either facilities, health workers or patients) are added to the chain since they would need to download all the data in blockchain to have an updated copy. This challenge is also a direct effect of the scalability issue in blockchain.

4. Security

Another implication of the property mentioned in the earlier challenge, is that since everyone has a copy of the blockchain, eventually it will be easier to hack on someone's blockchain copy. Instead of having a well-funded third party to attack, data hackers can hack on individual holders of blockchain records.

5. Data Protection Regulations

Many countries have adapt a data protection regulation pertaining to the right of individuals to request for a deletion/revision of their records stored in digital and non-digital media. Examples of these data protection regulations are the Data Protection

Act (Philippines) or the General Data Protection Regulation (GDPR) in Europe. These provisions are somehow opposite to blockchain's immutability property. Data protection regulation is seen as one of the biggest challenges to blockchain use.

Guide Questions:

(1) Are there technical work-around to the immutability property of blockchain versus the right to be deleted by persons?

Suggested Answers:

(1) Two possible ways of working around on this issue are

a. Participants don't store personal data in blockchain, but rather just use the chain as index to where the actual data are stored. Actual data may be stored in normal databases with CRUD functionalities.
b. Another possible workaround is the thrashing of data. Blockchain data are encrypted and if a person wants to delete or make his/her data useless, then a key destruction mechanism can be done, where the key that was used to encrypt the message will be destroyed, or be rendered useless. Once this is done, then the data stored in the blockchain will be practically unreadable.

7.5 Blockchain Use Cases in Health Care

In this section, three use cases of blockchain in Healthcare will be presented. For each use case, guide questions will be provided.

Use Case 1: Simple EHR Workflow

In a single health facility, all health transactions are uploaded to the blockchain. Using smart contracts, the designated personnel will be informed if a particular task is assigned to him. Example:

(1) Doctor X requests for an X-Ray on Patient Y from Radiologist Z.
(2) The request is stored in the blockchain
(3) Radiologist Z is informed that such a task is assigned to him.
(4) Radiologist Z performs an X-Ray on Patient Y
(5) Radiologist Z stores result of X-Ray in blockchain
(6) Doctor X is informed that the result is already available.

All the transactions are stored in the blockchain. Transactions are stored in the blockchain because there are many participants that are modifying the health/medical records of a patient.

Guide Questions:

(1) Who are the participants in the blockchain?
(2) What kind of blockchain design can be used?
(3) What are the potential issues in this design?

Suggested Answers:

(1) The participants of the blockchain are the different health providers in a facility. All participants should have a copy of the blockchain.
(2) A private/permissionless blockchain may be used since the health providers in the facility is a controlled population, and authentication credentials can be easily provided.
(3) The biggest issue with this design is that actual health data is stored in the blockchain. Another potential issue is scalability since all transactions done in the hospital will be recorded in the blockchain hence increasing its length.

Use Case 2: A Health Maintenance Organization (HMO) Claim Blockchain Workflow

In this workflow, there will be 5 identified transactions:

(1) Facility and HMO agrees to a contract of service
(2) Patient is enrolled in HMO
(3) Service is rendered by Facility to the Patient
(4) Facility makes a Claim from the HMO
(5) HMO pays claim.

Smart contracts can be assigned in the process. An example of smart contract use is to check whether there is an existing contract of service between the HMO and the Facility, and whether a patient is enrolled in an HMO, and whether service is provided to the patient, whenever a facility makes a claim from an HMO.

Guide Questions:

(1) Who are the participants in the blockchain?
(2) What kind of blockchain design can be used?
(3) What are the advantages of using blockchain in this workflow?
(4) What are the potential issues in this design?

Suggested Answers:

(1) The participants are the facilities, HMOs and the patients. Each may not need to have the contents of the whole blockchain (patients won't need the transaction nodes that are attributed from other patients).
(2) Since patients are participants, a public blockchain may be used. But since patients won't push data to the blockchain, it is possible that a permissionless blockchain is used since facilities and HMOs would need to be pre-registered/provided with authentication credentials before submitting data to the blockchain.
(3) Blockchain provides more sources of truth, and can be used offline. This is because all participants have a valid copy of the chain, it is easier to validate the truthfulness of transactions (rather than having a central entity to validate).
(4) Scalability will be a big issue since the chain will contain transactions by all patients in the locality,

Use Case 3: Design for a Patient Centric Health Information Exchange using Blockchain

In this workflow each patient will have his/her own blockchain recording all the transactions done in a health facility or with a healthcare provider. The blockchain will not store his/her health records, but rather it will only keep a pointer to the location of the associated health record. The health records will be kept in the Health facilities. Health facilities as participants in the blockchain will have a copy of the blockchains that are assigned to the patients.

Guide Questions:

(1) Who are the participants in the blockchain?
(2) What kind of blockchain design can be used?
(3) What are the potential issues in this design?
(4) Will the design scale up?

Suggested Answers:

(1) Patients, facilities (where the patients have been seen) are participants. Each patient has his/her own blockchain. Facilities have the blockchain of all patients that were seen in the facility.
(2) A private/permissionless blockchain may be used since each patient would be given credentials to his/her own blockchain, and facilities would have permissions when submitting data.
(3) The actual sharing of health data may be an issue since health data is not in the blockchain
(4) The design will scale up, since a blockchain will only increase in length, as a patient goes to a health facility. It is not expected that a lot of transactions will be stored in a chain since on average a person goes to a health facility only around 7 – 10 times a year. For each person, this amount of data is manageable.

7.6 Conclusion

Blockchain is seen as the most important technology that has been developed after the internet. It is set to change how data are stored and secured. As shown in this chapter, Healthcare is one of the areas that would benefit from blockchain. It has been discussed how the various properties of Healthcare use cases can fit into blockchain. But, despite the promises and the benefits of using blockchain, it is also quite noted that there are existing challenges. It is thus crucial that, before any blockchain solution is implemented, a suitable design and architecture phase must be first performed.

Acknowledgements SIL-Asia is powered by the Asia eHealth Information Network with support from the Asian Development Bank. The funds of the **laboratory** primarily came from the People's Republic of China Poverty Reduction and Regional Cooperation Fund. Additional support was provided by the World Health Organization, the Norwegian Aid Agency and UNICEF.

References

European Coordination Committee of the Radiological, Electromedical and Healthcare IT Industry. (2017). Beyond the hype of blockchain in healthcare, *COCIR*.

Haber, S., & Stornetta, W. (1991). How to time-stamp a digital document. *Journal of Cryptology, 3*.

Healthcare Data Breach Costs Higher than Any Industry. (2017). Retrieved February 20, 2019, from https://www.hipaajournal.com/healthcare-data-breach-costs-highest-of-any-industry-at-408-per-record/.

Nakamoto, S. (2008). Bitcoin a peer to peer electronic cash system. *Cryptography Mailing Lists.*

Zheng, Z., Xie, S., Dai, H.-N., Chen, X., & Wang, H. (2017). An overview of blockchain technology: Architecture. *Consensus, and Future Trends.* https://doi.org/10.1109/BigDataCongress.2017.85.

Part II
Applications of Data Science in Healthcare

8

Statistical Methods and their Usage in Python

Calvin J. Chiew

Abstract This chapter is based on a workshop I have conducted at several datathons introducing clinicians to popular statistical methods used in machine learning. It is primarily aimed at beginners who want a gentle, succinct guide to jumpstart their journey into practical machine learning and its applications in medicine. Thus, it is by no means a comprehensive guide on machine learning or Python. Rather, my hope is to present basic concepts in a simple, creative way, and demonstrate how they can be applied together.

Keywords Python · Crash course · Machine learning · Classification · Random forest · Support vector machine · Clinical prediction · Model fit · Cross-validation

Learning Objectives

- Readers will be able to run a simple program in Python
- Readers will be able to use a Jupyter Notebook
- Readers will understand basic concepts of supervised learning such as model fitting and cross-validation
- Readers will be able to differentiate between supervised learning methods for classification such as random forest and support vector machines

8.1 Introduction

A crash course on the basics of the Python language and Jupyter notebook environment will be presented in Sect. 8.2 to help those without prior programming experience get started quickly. You are welcome to skip this section if you are already familiar with Python. In Sects. 8.3, 8.4, 8.5, 8.6, I will introduce the random forest and support vector machine for classification, as well as general concepts of model fit and cross-validation. Finally, in a hands-on exercise in Sect. 8.7, you will be asked

C. J. Chiew (✉)
National University Health System, 1E Kent Ridge Rd, Singapore 119228, Singapore
e-mail: calvinjchiew@mail.harvard.edu

to implement and evaluate these models on a clinical prediction problem. Suggested solutions are provided for your reference. Each section ends with a summary that reinforces key concepts from that section. The corresponding files for this chapter can be found at https://github.com/criticaldata/globalhealthdatabook.git. If after reading this chapter you are motivated to learn more, there are plenty of print and online resources available (see Suggested Readings and References lists at the end).

8.1.1 Requirements & Setup Instructions

There are accompanying demos and exercises to this chapter which you are encouraged to access for the best educational experience. To do that, you will need a computer installed with **Python** and **Jupyter notebook**, the environment in which we will write and run Python code. By far the most convenient and reliable installation method is through the **Anaconda** distribution. This also comes with all the commonly used libraries or packages (i.e. the ones we need) bundled in, saving you the hassle of downloading and installing them one by one.

First, download the installer for Anaconda (Python 3 version) on your respective OS (Windows, Mac or Linux) from https://www.anaconda.com/download/. Then, run the installer and use all default options when prompted. Finally, after installation is complete, make sure you can open **Anaconda Navigator** and launch Jupyter notebook. (If you need help troubleshooting or have any programming-related questions, Stack Overflow [https://stackoverflow.com/] is a great place to look for answers.)

8.2 Python Crash Course

8.2.1 Terminology

Python is a programming language that has become popular for data science and machine learning (Guttag 2013). A **Jupyter notebook**, which is denoted by the file format `.ipynb`, is a document in which you can write and run Python code. It consists of cells, which can contain either Markdown (text) or code. Each cell can be executed independently, and the results of any code executed are "saved" until the file is closed. Raw data files are often **comma-separated values (CSV)** files which store tabular data in plain text. Each record consists of values (can be numeric or text) separated by commas. To see an example, open the accompanying dataset `births.csv` in Notepad and examine its contents. You can also open it in Excel for a tabular view.

There are many useful **libraries** or **modules** in Python which can be **imported** and **called** to make our lives easier and more convenient. SciPy is an ecosystem of Python libraries for math and science. The core libraries include NumPy, Pandas and Matplotlib. **NumPy** (typically imported as `np`) allows you to work efficiently with data in arrays. **Pandas** (typically imported as `pd`) can load csv data into **dataframes** which optimize storage and manipulation of data. Dataframes have useful methods such as `head`, `shape`, `merge` etc. The **pyplot** module (typically imported as `plt`) in **matplotlib** contains useful functions for generating simple plots e.g. `plot`, `scatter`, `hist` etc. You will encounter these libraries and their functions in the demo and hands-on exercise later.

8.2.2 Basic Built-in Data Types

The basic built-in data types you should be familiar with in Python are **integer, float, Boolean, string** and **list**. Examples of each type are as follows:

Integer	`7`
Float	`7.0`
Boolean	`True, False`
String	`'Hi', "7.0"`
List	`[], ['Hello', 70, 2.1, True]`

Strings can be enclosed by either single or double quotation marks. Lists are collections of items, which can be of different types. They are indicated by square brackets, with items separated by commas. Unlike older programming languages like C, you do not need to declare the types of your variables in Python. The type is inferred from the value assigned to the variable.

8.2.3 Python Demo

You do not need to be a Python expert in order to use it for machine learning. The best way to learn Python is simply to practice using it on several datasets. In line with this philosophy, let us review the basics of Python by seeing it in action.

Open Anaconda Navigator and launch Jupyter Notebook. In the browser that pops up, navigate to the folder where you have saved the accompanying files to this chapter. Click on `demo.ipynb`. In this notebook, there are a series of cells containing small snippets of Python code. Clicking the "play" button (or hitting Shift + Enter) will execute the currently selected (highlighted) cell. Run through each cell in this demo one by one—see if you understand what the code means and whether the output matches what you expect. Can you identify the data type of each variable.

In cell 1, the * operator represents multiplication and in cell 2, the == operator represents equality. In cell 3, we create a list of 3 items and assign it to `lst` with the = operator. Note that when cell 3 is executed, there is no output, but the value of `lst` is saved in the kernel's memory. That is why when we index into the first item of `lst` in cell 4, the kernel already knows about `lst` and does not throw an error.

Indexing into a list or string is done using square brackets. Unlike some other programming languages, Python is **zero-indexed**, i.e. counting starts from zero, not one! Therefore, in cells 4 and 5, we use `[0]` and `[1:]` to indicate that we want the first item, and the second item onwards, respectively.

In cell 6, we ask for the length of `lst` with the built-in **function** `len()`. In cell 7, we create a **loop** with the `for`...`in`... construct, printing a line for each iteration of the loop with `print()`. Note that the number '5' is not printed even though we stated `range(5)`, demonstrating again that Python starts counting from zero, not one.

In cell 8, we define our own function `add()` with the `def` and `return` keywords. There is again no output here but the definition of `add()` is saved once we execute this cell. We then call our function `add()` in cell 9, giving it two inputs (arguments) 1 and 2, and obtaining an output of 3 as expected.

In cell 10, we define a more complicated function `rate()` which when given a letter grade (as a string), outputs a customized string. We create branches within this function with the `if`...`elif`...`else` construct. One important thing to note here is the use of **indentation** to indicate nesting of code. Proper indentation is non-negotiable in Python. Code blocks are not indicated by delimiters such as `{}`, only by indentation. If indentation is incorrect (for example if this block of code were written all flushed to the left), the kernel would throw an error. In cells 11 and 12, we call our function `rate()` and check that we obtain desired outputs as expected.

Taking a step back, notice how Python syntax is close to plain English. Code readability is important for us to maintain code (imagine coming back 6 months later and realizing you cannot make sense of your own code!) as well as for others to understand our work.

It is not possible (nor necessary) to cover everything about Python in this crash course. Below I have compiled a list of common operators and keywords into a "cheat sheet" for beginners.

Arithmetic	`+, -, *, /, %, **, //`
Comparison	`== , != , > , < , >=, <=`
Boolean logic	`and, or, not`
Indexing lists/strings	`[n], [n:m], [n:], [:n]`
Selection	`if, elif, else`
Iteration/loop	`for, in, range`
Create function	`def, return`
Call function	`function(arg1, arg2, …)`
Call object's method or library's function	`object.method(arg1, arg2, …)` `library.function(arg1, arg2, …)`
Get length of list/string	`len(…)`
Import library	`import … as …`
Print	`print()`

8.2.4 *Python Exercise*

You are now ready to practice your Python skills. Open the notebook `python.ipynb` and give the exercise a shot. In this exercise, we will practice some simple data exploration, which is an important aspect of the data science process before model-building. Try to give your variables descriptive names (e.g. "age", "gender" are preferable to "a", "b"). If you are stuck, refer to `python_solutions.ipynb` for suggested solutions. Read on for more explanations.

In the very first cell, we import the libraries we need (e.g. pandas) and give them short names (e.g. `pd`) so that we can refer to them easily later. In Q1, we read in the dataset into a pandas dataframe `births` by calling the `read_csv()` function from `pd`. Note that the data file `births.csv` should be in the same folder as the notebook, otherwise you have to specify its location path. `births` is a dataframe **object** and we can call its **methods** `head` and `shape` (using the `object.method` notation) to print its first 5 rows and its dimensions. Note that the shape of dataframes is always given as (number of rows, number of columns). In this case, we have 400 rows and 3 columns.

It is worth spending some time at this juncture to clarify how we index into 2D arrays such as dataframes, since it is something we commonly need to do. The element at the n-th row and the m-th column is indexed as [n, m]. Just like lists, you can get multiple array values at a time. Look at the figures below and convince yourself that we can index into the blue elements of each 2D array by the following commands. Remember, Python is zero-indexed.

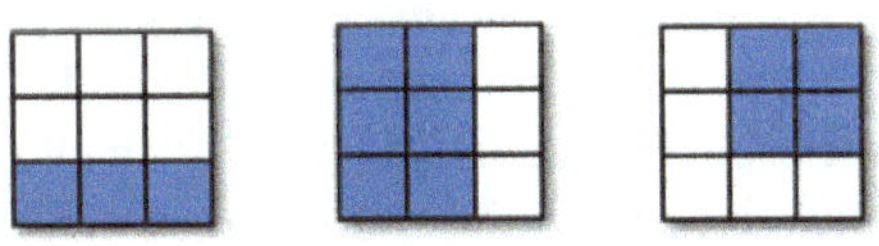

`arr[2]` `arr[2, :]` `arr[:, :2]` `arr[:2, 1:]`

In Q2, we call the `mean` method to quickly obtain the mean value for each column in `births`. In Q3, we create 3 copies of the `births` dataframe—`group1`, `group2` and `group3`. For each group, we select (filter) the rows we want from `births` based on maternal age. Note the use of operators to specify the logic. We then apply `shape` and `mean` methods again to obtain the number of births and mean birth weight for each group and `print()` them out.

In Q4, we call `scatter()` from the `pyplot` module (which we have earlier imported as `plt`) to draw a scatterplot of data from `births`, specifying `birth_weight` as the x-axis, and `femur_length` as the y-axis. Note the use of `figure()` to start an empty figure, `xlabel()` and `ylabel()` to specify the axis labels, and `show()` to print the figure.

The code in Q5 is similar, except that we call `scatter()` 3 times, using data from `group1`, `group2` and `group3` instead of `births`, and specifying the different colors we want for each group. We use `legend()` to also include a key explaining the colors and their labels in the figure. If we wanted to add a figure title, we could have done that with `title()`.

8.3 Model Fit

In machine learning, we are often interested in prediction. Given a set of **predictors** or **features** (X1, X2, X3...), we want to predict the **response** or **outcome** (Y). Mathematically speaking, we want to estimate f in $Y = f(X_1, X_2, X_3 \ldots) + \varepsilon$, where f is a function of our predictors and ε is some error. (James et al. 2013) If Y is a continuous variable, we call this task **regression**. If Y is categorical, we call it **classification**.

We choose an **error** or **loss function** that is appropriate for the prediction task. In regression, we commonly use mean squared error (MSE), which is the sum of residuals squared divided by sample size. In classification, the error can simply be the number of misclassifications.

Data is typically split into two distinct subsets—**training** and **testing**. The training set is used to create the model, i.e. estimate f. The testing set is used to evaluate the model, i.e. to see how good f is at predicting Y given a set of X. Therefore, the testing set acts as an independent, fair judge of our model's performance. The size of the train-test split is dependent on the size and specifics of the dataset, although it is common to use 60–80% of the data for training and the remainder for testing.

Both the training and testing error will decrease up to a point of optimum model fit (dotted line). Beyond that, **overfitting** occurs as the model becomes more specific to the training data, and less generalizable (flexible) to the testing data. Even though the training error continues to decline, the testing error starts to go up. Another way to think of overfitting is that an overfitted model picks up the "noise" of the function rather than focusing on the "signals". It is thus important for us to separate data into training and testing sets from the start, so that we can detect overfitting and avoid it.

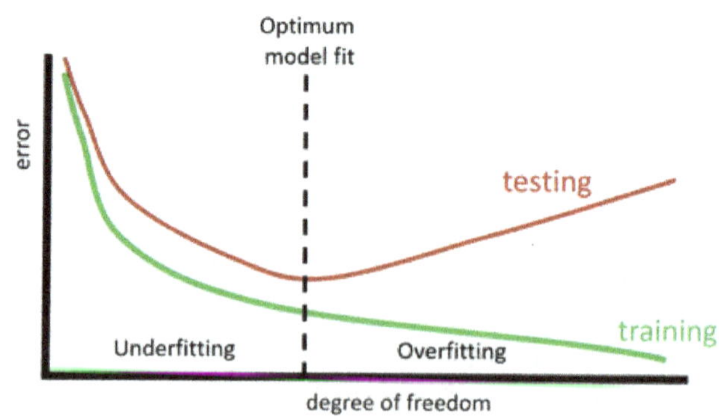

Summary

- In statistical modelling, we want to estimate f in Y = f(X) + e, where Y is the response (outcome), X is a set of features (predictors), and e is the error.
- To prevent overfitting, we split the data into training and testing sets. We develop the model on the training set, then evaluate its performance on the testing set.
- We choose an error (loss) function appropriate for the prediction task, e.g. mean squared error for regression (continuous Y), sum of misclassifications for classification (categorical Y).

8.4 Random Forest

8.4.1 Decision Tree

A **decision tree** is simply a series of splitting or **branching** rules. Take a look at this decision tree which predicts whether a patient walking into the Emergency Room with chest pain has Acute Myocardial Infarction (AMI), commonly known as "heart attack".

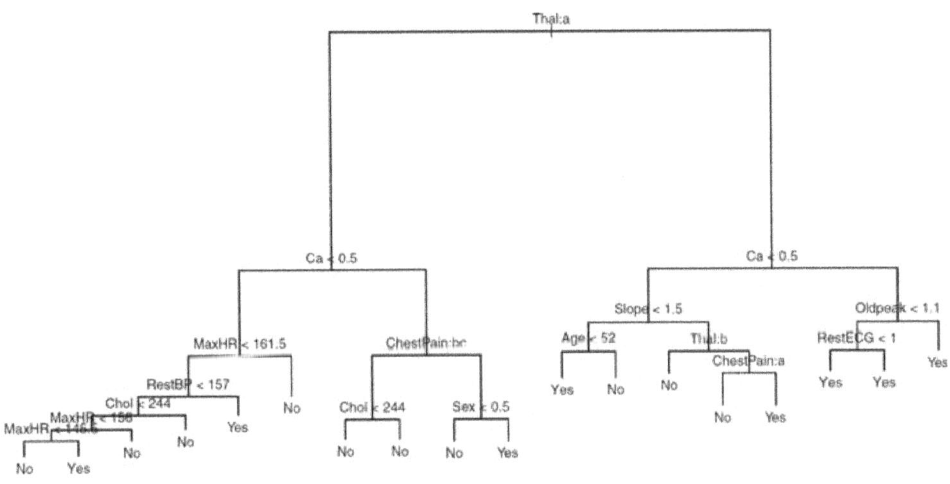

We start from the top and move our way down the tree. At each branching point or **node**, we either go left or right depending on whether the patient meets the criteria specified. For example, at the first branch, we go left if the patient is < 50 years old, or right if the patient is $\geq$ 50 years old. Each branch features one predictor, for example age, blood pressure, heart rate or cholesterol. The same predictor can appear multiple times in the tree and with different thresholds. Eventually, we reach the bottom, in one of the **terminal nodes** or **leaves**, where we obtain a prediction—either yes or no. A decision tree is thus very easy to visualize and understand.

To build the tree, an algorithm called **recursive binary splitting** is used. While the underlying mathematical theory of this algorithm is beyond the scope of this chapter, we can think of it at a conceptual level. In the case of a classification tree here, the algorithm aims to increase **node purity**, indicated by a lower **Gini index**, with each successive split. This means we want observations that fall into each node to be predominantly from the same class. Intuitively, we understand why—if the majority (or all) of the observations in one node are "yes", then we are quite confident any future observation that follows the same branching pattern into that node will also be a "yes".

Since the branching can continue infinitely, we must specify a stopping criterion, for example until each terminal node has some minimum number of observations (minimum node size), or a certain maximum tree depth is reached. Note that it is possible to split a node into two leaves with the same predicted class, if doing so achieves higher node purity (creates more certainty).

8.4.2 Random Forest

A **random forest**, as the name suggests, contains multiple decision trees. It is an example of the **ensemble** method, a commonly used machine learning technique of combining many models to achieve one optimal model. A disadvantage of decision trees is that they have high variance, that is if we change the training data by a little bit, we get a very different looking tree, so the result is not stable. To deal with this, we want to produce multiple trees and then take the **majority vote** of their predictions to reduce uncertainty.

We get that many trees form a forest, but why random? If we train all the trees the same way, they are all going to learn the same thing—all of them will choose the most important predictor as the top branch, and the next important predictor as the second branch, and so forth. We will end up with trees that are just clones of each other, defeating our original intent. What we really want are trees that can complement each other's weaknesses and errors. To harness the "power of crowds", we need diversity, not herd mentality.

Thus, at each branching point, only a **random subset** of all the predictors are considered as potential split candidates. Doing so enables us to get trees that are less similar to each other, obtaining a random forest.

In a random forest, feature importance can be visualized by calculating the total decrease in Gini index due to splits over each predictor, averaged over all trees. The following graph shows the relative importance of each feature in a random forest model predicting AMI in patients with chest pain from earlier.

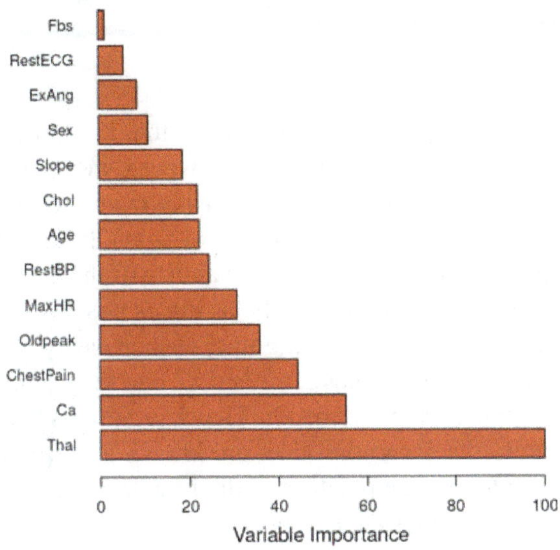

Summary

- Random forest is an ensemble method combining multiple decision trees to improve prediction accuracy.
- A decision tree is essentially a series of branching rules based on the predictors.
- To build a classification tree, we use recursive binary splitting, and aim to increase node purity with each split. A stopping criterion is specified, e.g. minimum node size, maximum tree depth.
- At each branching point, only a random subset of all predictors are considered as potential split candidates. This is done to decorrelate the trees.

8.5 Support Vector Machine

8.5.1 Maximal Margin Classifier

Imagine we have only two predictors, x1 and x2, and we plot our training observations on a graph of x2 against x1 as follows. Now if asked to draw a line that separates the two classes (yellow and blue), where would you draw it?

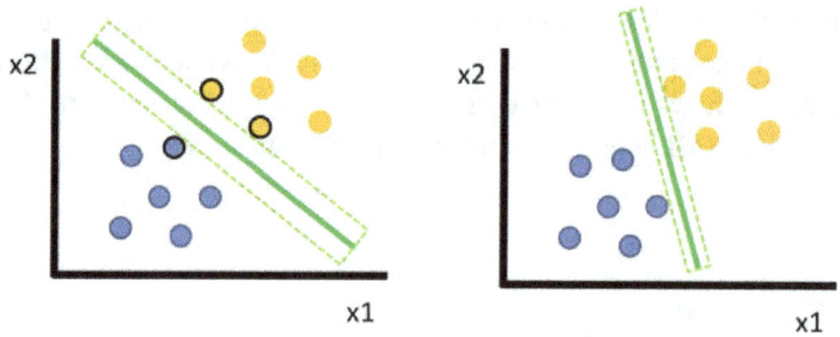

There are in fact infinitely many possible lines that could be drawn to separate the yellow and blue observations in this case. However, we naturally tend to draw a line with the largest **margin**—the one furthest away from the training observations (i.e. we prefer the line on the left to the one on the right). Intuitively, we understand why—the margin reflects our confidence in the ability of the line to separate the two classes. Therefore, we want this margin to be as big as possible.

Once we have determined the separating line, we can easily predict the class of a test observation, by plugging its values of x1 and x2 into the equation of the line, and see if we obtain a positive or negative result. The observations that lie on the margin (dashed box), closest to the separating line, are known as **support vectors** (points with black outline). Note that the position of the line depends solely on the support vectors. If we erase all the other data points, we will still end up drawing the same line. In this way, the other data points are redundant to obtaining the solution.

We can extend this basic premise to situations where there are more than two predictors. When there are 3 predictors, the data points are now in a 3-dimensional space, and the separating line becomes a separating plane. When there are p predictors, the data points are in a p-dimensional space, and so we now have a (p-1)-dimensional **separating hyperplane**.

8.5.2 Support Vector Classifier

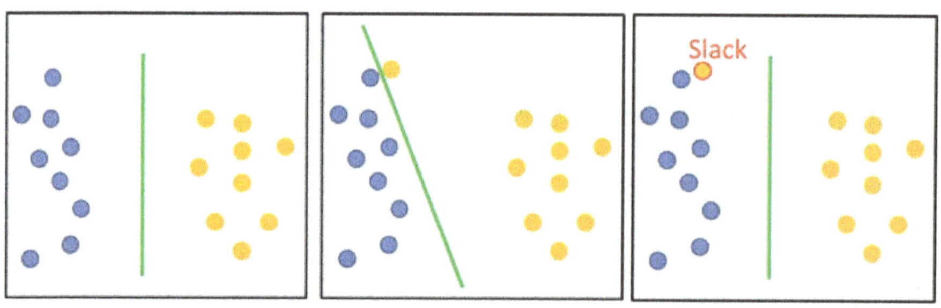

Now imagine we have an outlier in the yellow group, which causes the position of the separating line to shift dramatically (second box). We are uncomfortable with this new line because it has been unduly influenced by a single data point and is probably not generalizable to the testing data. Ideally, we want the line to remain in its original position, ignoring the outlier (third box). To achieve this, we allow some "**slack**" for data points to be on the "wrong" side of the hyperplane in exchange for a more robust hyperplane against outliers.

The tuning parameter 'C' controls the amount of slack—when C is small, more slack is allowed (more tolerant of wrongly classified points), resulting in a softer (but wider) margin. The value of 'C' is usually chosen by cross-validation (see Sect. 8.6).

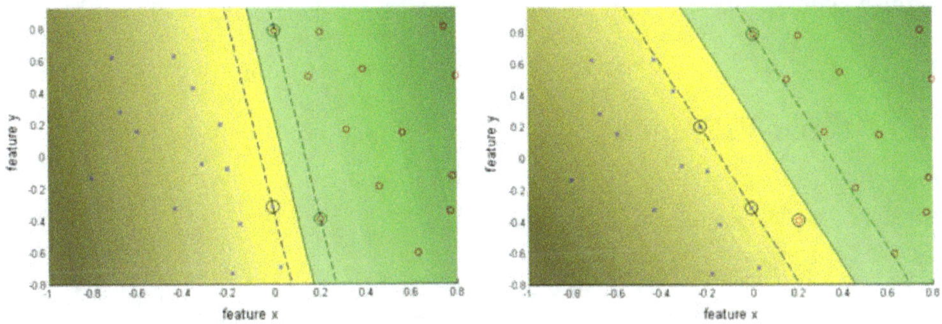

Hard margin (large C) (left); soft margin (small C) (right)

Given a set of data points that are not linearly separable on the input space, we can use a **kernel function** Φ to project them onto a higher-dimensional feature space and draw the linear separating hyperplane in that space. When projected back onto the input space, the decision boundary is non-linear. The kernel function can also be chosen by cross-validation (see Sect. 8.6), or commonly the radial basis function (RBF) kernel is used.

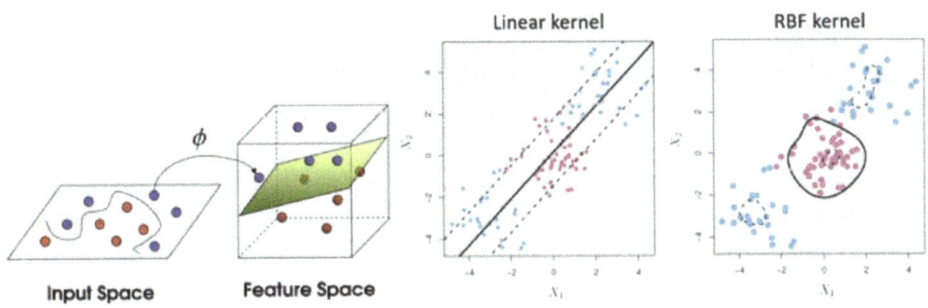

Summary

- In SVM, we want to draw a (p-1)-dimensional separating hyperplane between the classes, where p is the number of predictors.
- If multiple hyperplanes are possible, we choose the one with the largest margin.
- To make the separating hyperplane more robust to outliers, we tolerate some observations on the wrong side of the hyperplane. The tuning parameter C controls the amount of slack given. A smaller C results in a softer margin.

- Given a set of data points that are not linearly separable, we can use a non-linear kernel function (e.g. radial basis function, RBF) to project them onto a higher-dimensional space and draw the separating hyperplane in that space.

8.6 Miscellaneous Topics

In this section, we will cover 3 more concepts that are important for the hands-on exercise later.

8.6.1 Cross-Validation

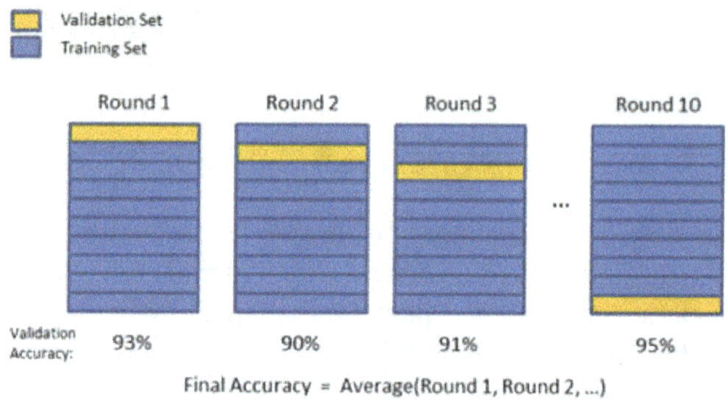

Cross-validation (CV) is a method of resampling often used to choose (tune) parameters of a model. We should not arbitrarily choose model parameters ourselves if we cannot justify or defend these choices that may impact model performance. CV helps us to make the best choices that maximize model performance based on the available data.

In k-fold CV, we split the *training* data into k folds, take one fold to validate and remaining k-1 folds to train. We then calculate a chosen performance metric (e.g. accuracy or error rate), repeat k times and take the average result. Note that we do not touch the independent set of testing data until the model is complete for evaluation.

Examples of parameters that could be tuned for a random forest model are the number of trees, the number of predictors considered at each split and the maximum tree depth or minimum node size. Examples of parameters that could be tuned for a SVM model are the amount of slack tolerated (C), the kernel and kernel coefficient. Before building any model, check the library's documentation to see what tuning parameters are available.

When there are two or more parameters we wish to tune concurrently (e.g. number of trees *and* maximum tree depth for a random forest), we can turn to **Grid Search CV**. We first define the range of candidate values for each parameter through which the algorithm should search. The algorithm then performs CV on all possible combinations of parameters to find the best set of parameters for our chosen evaluation metric.

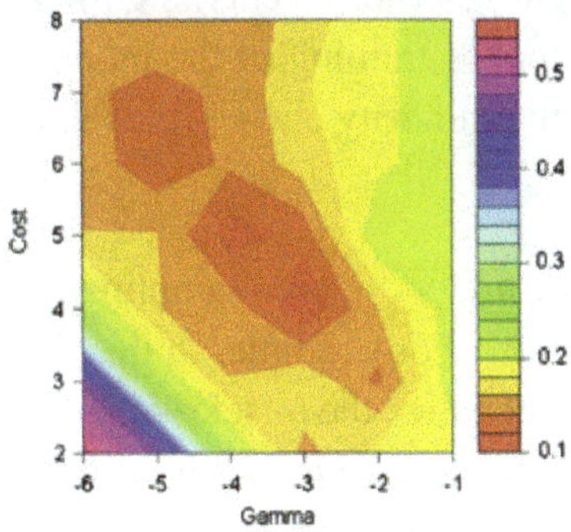

8.6.2 Receiver Operating Characteristic (ROC) Curve

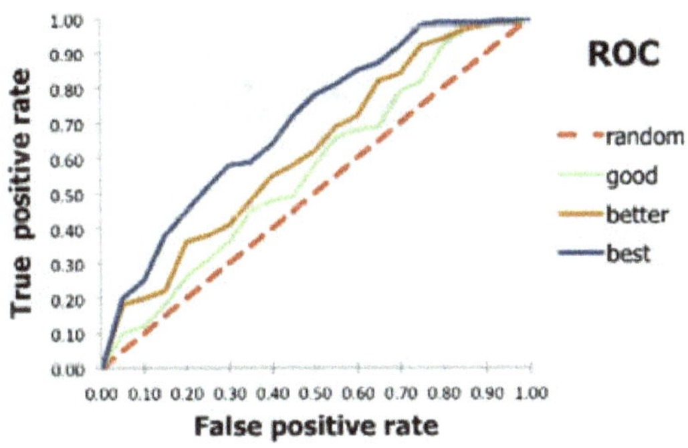

Receiver Operating Characteristic (ROC) curves are often used to evaluate and compare the performance of various models. It is a plot of true positive rate (sensitivity) against false positive rate (1-specificity), and illustrates the trade-off between sensitivity and specificity. Sensitivity refers to the proportion of positives that are correctly classified as positive (true positive rate), while specificity refers to the proportion of negatives that are correctly classified as negative (true negative rate). The overall performance of a classifier is given by the **area under the curve (AUC)**. An ideal ROC curve will hug the top left corner of the graph, maximizing the AUC. Random guessing is equivalent to AUC of 0.5.

8.6.3 *Imbalanced Data*

It is quite common to encounter **imbalanced datasets** in medicine, where most of the samples belong to one class, with very few samples from the other class. Usually, the number of negatives (non-events) significantly outweighs the number of positives (events). This makes training of the models difficult, as there is sparse data to learn how to detect the minority class, which tends to get "overwhelmed" by the majority class.

Possible solutions include under- or over-sampling to create balanced datasets, or re-weighting the sample points. For example, in this SVM model, if **class weights** are applied (dotted line), we penalize the misclassification of the minority class (red) more than the majority class (blue), i.e. we sacrifice the majority class to prioritize the correct classification of the minority class. In doing so, we obtain a better separating hyperplane than if class weights were not applied (solid line).

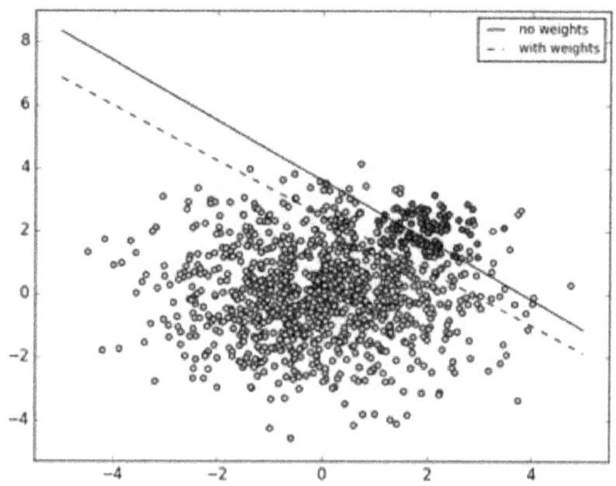

Summary

- Cross-validation is a resampling method that can be used to tune parameters of a model.
- In k-fold CV, we split the training data into k folds, take one fold to validate and remaining k-1 folds to train. Then calculate the chosen performance metric, repeat k times and average the result.
- A Receiver Operating Characteristic (ROC) curve is a plot of true positive rate (sensitivity) against false positive rate. An ideal classifier will produce a curve that hugs the top left-hand corner, maximizing the area under the curve (AUC). Random guessing is equivalent to AUC of 0.5.
- When dealing with imbalanced data, we can under- or over-sample to create balanced datasets, or apply class weights.

8.7 Hands-on Exercise

8.7.1 Sample Code Review

Let us now review some sample code for a simple machine learning project together. Open the notebook `sample.ipynb`. The premise for this project is described at the top.

We begin by importing the libraries we need, the most important of which is `sklearn`, a library for machine learning containing functions for creating various statistical models and other useful functions (Geron 2017). The code in this sample is interspersed with **comments**, indicated by #, explaining what each code block does.

In the Data Preparation section, we load the dataset into `data` with `read_csv()` and check its `head` and `shape` to make sure they match what we expect (see Sect. 8.2.4 if this is unfamiliar to you). We then split `data` into the predictor variables (named `x`) and response variable (named `y`) using its `values` method and appropriate indexing (see Sect. 8.2.4 for more help). Again, we perform a sanity check on the shapes of `x` and `y`. Next, we feed `x` and `y` into the `train_test_split()` function from `sklearn` to split our data into training and testing sets. The argument `test_size = 0.3` indicates that we want to use 30% of the observations for testing, with the remaining 70% for training. The `random_state = 123` argument indicates the seed for the random number generator. Fixing the seed (any random number is okay) ensures that we obtain the same train-test split every time for reproducibility. If this argument was not specified, we would obtain different train-test splits each time this code is executed. Lastly, we perform sanity checks again—we have 773 samples in the training set and 332 samples in the testing set. In both sets, more patients have benign tumour than malignant cancer, so we have some imbalanced data.

In the Model Building section, we see that it is in fact very simple to create the models using `sklearn`. We instantiate two objects `rf` and `svm` by calling `RandomForestClassifier()` and `SVC()` from `sklearn` respectively. Then, we `fit()` them with the training data. The `class_weight='balanced'` argument indicates that we want to apply class weights to address class imbalance. The `n_estimators = 30` argument for the random forest (RF) model indicates the number of trees in the forest. The `kernel='linear'` argument for the support vector machine (SVM) model indicates a linear kernel function (as opposed to RBF for example). We have defined a custom `score()` function, which when given a model and testing data, uses the model's innate `score` method to calculate its overall test accuracy, specificity and sensitivity. Lastly, we present all the scores neatly in a dataframe. Both models have similar test accuracies (RF 83%, SVM 85%). The RF model has higher specificity (90% vs. 87%) while the SVM model has higher sensitivity (82% vs. 73%).

In the Parameter Tuning section, we use grid search cross-validation to find the best maximum depth of trees for the RF model and best C parameter for the SVM model. We define the parameters and range of candidate values to search in `parameters`. (Increasing the range and granularity of our search would be more thorough but at the expense of computation time.) We then input the model and `parameters` to the function `GridSearchCV()`. The `cv = 5` argument indicates that we want to use 5 folds for cross-validation. `GridSearchCV()` returns the tuned model which we `fit()` and `score()` again. We see that after tuning, both models perform slightly better (overall test accuracies RF 85%, SVM 86%). The best `max_depth` was determined to be 6 and the best `C` was 0.1.

In the Model Evaluation section, we use the tuned models to generate predicted probabilities on the testing data, and input them with the true outcome (y) labels into `roc_curve()` to obtain a series of true positive rates (`tpr`) and corresponding false positive rates (`fpr`). We then graph these `tpr` and `fpr` using the `plot()` function from `pyplot`, forming ROC curves. `auc()` is used to calculate the area under the curve for each model. We see that the ROC curves and AUC for both models are similar (RF 0.91, SVM 0.92).

In addition, we visualize the top 5 most predictive features and their relative importance in the RF model. We do this by calling the `feature_importances_` method from the `rf` model, which returns the importance of each feature based on the total decrease in Gini index method described in Sect. 8.4.2. We sort them in order and obtain the indices of the last five (with highest importances). We then match them to column names from `data` based on their indices. Finally, we graph the information on a horizontal bar plot using `barh()` from `pyplot`.

8.7.2 Hands-on Exercise

You are now ready to apply all that you have learnt! Complete the questions in `exercise.ipynb`. You may adapt code from `sample.ipynb` as a template, but you will need to make necessary changes as appropriate. Copying-and-pasting without understanding will most certainly lead to errors! When you are done, check your answers against the suggested solutions in `solutions.ipynb`.

I hope this chapter has been a useful introduction to machine learning and to programming in Python for those who are new. We have barely just scratched the surface of this vast, exciting field. Indeed, there are many more modelling techniques beyond random forest and support vector machine which we have discussed here. The table below lists some of the popular algorithms currently. You should have sufficient foundation now to explore on your own. Many of these methods are implemented in `sklearn` and you can Google the documentation for them. The best way to make all of this come alive is to design and implement your own machine learning project that is of interest and value to you or your organization.

Supervised Learning	*Unsupervised Learning*
• K-nearest neighbours • Regression (linear, logistic, polynomial, spline etc.) ± regularization • Linear/quadratic discriminant analysis • Tree-based approaches: decision tree, bagging, random forest, boosting • Support vector machine • Neural network	• Principal components analysis • Clustering • Neural network

References

Géron, A. (2017). Hands-on machine learning with scikit-learn and tensorflow: concepts, tools, and techniques to build intelligent systems. O'Reilly Media.

Guttag, J. (2013). Introduction to computation and programming using Python. The MIT Press.

James, G., Witten, D., Hastie, T., & Tibshirani, R. (2013). An introduction to statistical learning with applications in R. Springer.

9

Machine Learning for Phenotyping: Data Preparation and Analysis

Cátia M. Salgado and Susana M. Vieira

Abstract Machine Learning for Phenotyping is composed of three chapters and aims to introduce clinicians to machine learning (ML). It provides a guideline through the basic concepts underlying machine learning and the tools needed to easily implement it using the Python programming language and Jupyter notebook documents. It is divided into three main parts: part 1—data preparation and analysis; part 2—unsupervised learning for clustering, and part 3—supervised learning for classification.

Keywords Machine learning · Phenotyping · Data preparation · Data analysis · Unsupervised learning · Clustering · Supervised learning · Classification · Clinical informatics

9.1 Learning Objectives and Approach

It is recommended that you follow this chapter using the jupyter notebook provided in https://github.com/cmsalgado/book_chapter, so that you can experiment with the code on your own. Since we are not implementing most of the algorithms and models, you will be able to follow the notebook even if you have no prior experience with coding. We will cover a large number of well-known ML algorithms, starting with the simplest (logistic regression and k-nearest neighbors) and ending with more complex ones (random forest), without delving in much detail into the underlying mathematical theory. Instead, we will focus on explaining the intuitions behind algorithms so that you understand how they learn and how you can use and interpret them for any new problem.

A real-world clinical dataset will be used. It was constructed based on the code provided in https://github.com/YerevaNN/mimic3-benchmarks for the prediction of hospital mortality using data collected during the first two days in the ICU. The data was extracted from the MIMIC-III Clinical Database, which is a large,

---

C. M. Salgado (✉) · S. M. Vieira
IDMEC Instituto Superior Técnico, Universidade de Lisboa, Av. Rovisco Pais, Lisboa, Portugal
e-mail: catia.salgado@tecnico.ulisboa.pt

publicly-available database comprising de-identified electronic health records of approximately 60 000 ICU admissions. Patients stayed in the intensive care unit (ICU) of the Beth Israel Deaconess Medical Center between 2001 and 2012. MIMIC-III database is described in:

Johnson AEW, Pollard TJ, Shen L, Lehman L, Feng M, Ghassemi M, Moody B, Szolovits P, Celi LA, Mark RG. MIMIC-III, a freely accessible critical care database. Scientific Data (2016).

Before dwelling into ML, this chapter presents the data preparation phase, which consists of a series of steps required to transform raw data from electronic health records into structured data that can be used as input to the learning algorithms. This is a crucial part of any ML project. First, it is important to understand what the algorithm is supposed to learn so that you can select appropriate information/variables to describe the problem. In other words, you want to avoid what is frequently referred to as "garbage in, garbage out". Second, since it is usually not handed in a format that is ready for straightaway ML, chances are that you will need to spend some time preprocessing and analyzing the data. You will see that in the end, your results are highly dependent on decisions made during this part. It does not matter to keep trying to optimize the ML algorithm if you have poor data, your algorithm will not be able to learn. In this scenario, you probably gain more by going back to the stages of data extraction and preprocessing and rethink your decisions; it is better to have good data and a simple algorithm than poor data and a very complex algorithm. In particular, the data preparation phase consists of:

- Exploratory data analysis
- Variable selection
- Identification and exclusion of outliers
- Data aggregation
- Inclusion criteria
- Feature construction
- Data partitioning.

The machine learning phase consists of:

- Patient stratification through unsupervised learning
  - k-means clustering
- Patient classification through supervised learning
  - Feature selection
  - Logistic regression
  - Decision trees
  - Random forest.

9.2 Prerequisites

In order to run the code provided in this Chapter, you should have Python and the following Python libraries installed:

- NumPy: fundamental package for scientific computing with Python. Provides a fast numerical array structure.
- Pandas: provides high-performance, easy-to-use data structures and data analysis tools.
- Scikit-learn: essential machine learning package in Python. Provides simple and efficient tools for data mining and data analysis.
- matplotlib: basic plotting library.
- seaborn: visualization library based on matplotlib. It provides a high-level interface for drawing statistical graphics.
- IPython: for interactive data visualization.
- Jupyter: for interactive computing.

It is highly recommended that you install Anaconda, which already has the above packages and more included. Additionally, in order to be able to visualize decision trees, you should install pydot and graphviz. Next, we will import the python libraries that we will need for now and MIMIC-III data.

9.2.1 Import Libraries and Data

The next example shows the Python code that imports Numpy, Pandas, Matplotlib and IPython libraries:

```
In [1]: import numpy as np
         import pandas as pd
         import matplotlib.pyplot as plt
         from IPython import display
         import warnings


         plt.style.use('ggplot')
```

The next example shows the Python code that loads the data as a Pandas DataFrame, which is a tabular data structure that makes it easy to do all kinds of manipulations such as arithmetic operations and grouping. The unique ICU stay ID is used as the DataFrame index, for facilitating data manipulation. This is achived by setting the 'index_col' parameter to the name of the index column.

```
In [2]: data = pd.read_csv('/https://www.dropbox.com/s/3l20njo1sb5ui4g/mimic3_mortality.csv?raw=1_',
    index_col='icustay')
```

9.3 Exploratory Data Analysis

A quick preview of 'data' can be obtained using the 'head' function, which prints the first 5 rows of any given DataFrame:

```
In [3]: data.head()
```

```
Out[3]:           hours  diastolic BP  glasgow coma scale  glucose  heart rate  \
icustay
282372.0  0.066667          60.0                 NaN      NaN       139.0
282372.0  0.150000          73.0                 NaN      NaN       128.0
282372.0  0.233333          81.0                 NaN      NaN       127.0
282372.0  0.316667          86.0                 NaN      NaN       132.0
282372.0  0.400000          86.0                 NaN      NaN       138.0

             mean BP  oxygen saturation  respiratory rate  systolic BP  \
icustay
282372.0   84.666702              100.0              20.0        134.0
282372.0   93.000000              100.0              25.0        133.0
282372.0   88.666702              100.0              22.0        104.0
282372.0  100.000000              100.0              19.0        128.0
282372.0  100.333000              100.0              21.0        129.0

          temperature        age  gender  height  pH  weight  day  mortality
icustay
282372.0          NaN  48.682393     2.0     NaN NaN    59.0    1          1
282372.0          NaN  48.682393     2.0     NaN NaN    59.0    1          1
282372.0          NaN  48.682393     2.0     NaN NaN    59.0    1          1
282372.0          NaN  48.682393     2.0     NaN NaN    59.0    1          1
282372.0          NaN  48.682393     2.0     NaN NaN    59.0    1          1
```

It tells us that the dataset contains information regarding patient demographics: age, gender, weight, height, mortality; physiological vital signs: diastolic blood pressure, systolic blood pressure, mean blood pressure, temperature, respiratory rate; lab tests: glucose, pH; scores: glasgow coma scale. Each observation/row is associated with a time stamp (column 'hours'), indicating the number of hours since ICU admission where the observation was made. Each icustay has several observations for the same variable/column.

We can print the number of ICU stays by calculating the length of the unique indexes, number of missing data using the 'info' function and summary statistics using the 'describe' function:

```
In [4]: print('Number of ICU stays: ' + str(len(data.index.unique())))
        print('Number of survivors: ' + str(len(data[data['mortality']==0].index.unique())))
        print('Number of non-survivors: ' + str(len(data[data['mortality']==1].index.unique())))
        print('Mortality: ' + str(round(100*len(data[data['mortality']==1].index.unique()) /
        len(data.index.unique()),1)) + '%')
        print()
        display.display(data.info(null_counts=1))
        display.display(data.describe())
```

```
Number of ICU stays: 21139
Number of survivors: 18342
Number of non--survivors: 2797
Mortality: 13.2%
```

```
<class 'pandas.core.frame.DataFrame'>
Float64Index: 1461282 entries, 282372.0 to 245756.0
Data columns (total 18 columns):
hours                   1461282 non-null float64
diastolic BP            1015241 non-null float64
glasgow coma scale      159484 non-null float64
glucose                 248460 non-null float64
heart rate              1057551 non-null float64
mean BP                 1007986 non-null float64
oxygen saturation       1065406 non-null float64
respiratory rate        1066675 non-null float64
systolic BP             1015683 non-null float64
temperature             321762 non-null float64
age                     1461282 non-null float64
gender                  1461282 non-null float64
height                  455361 non-null float64
pH                      116414 non-null float64
weight                  1309930 non-null float64
day                     1461282 non-null int64
mortality               1461282 non-null int64
hour                    1461282 non-null float64
dtypes: float64(16), int64(2)
memory usage: 251.8 MB
```

```
              hours  diastolic BP  glasgow coma scale        glucose  \
count  1.461282e+06  1.015241e+06       159484.000000  248460.000000
mean   2.182227e+01  6.031228e+01           11.600668     143.930140
std    1.421245e+01  1.452069e+01            3.920855      67.442769
min    0.000000e+00 -1.300000e+01            3.000000       0.000000
25%    8.938958e+00  5.100000e+01            9.000000     106.000000
50%    2.091528e+01  5.900000e+01           14.000000     129.000000
75%    3.404250e+01  6.800000e+01           15.000000     162.000000
max    4.800000e+01  2.980000e+02           15.000000    1748.000000

         heart rate       mean BP  oxygen saturation  respiratory rate  \
count  1.057551e+06  1.007986e+06       1.065406e+06      1.066675e+06
mean   8.697399e+01  7.831875e+01       9.678339e+01      1.920545e+01
std    1.886481e+01  1.627105e+01       4.695637e+00      6.246538e+00
min    0.000000e+00  0.000000e+00       0.000000e+00      0.000000e+00
25%    7.400000e+01  6.700000e+01       9.600000e+01      1.500000e+01
50%    8.500000e+01  7.600000e+01       9.800000e+01      1.900000e+01
75%    9.900000e+01  8.700000e+01       1.000000e+02      2.300000e+01
max    3.000000e+02  3.000000e+02       1.000000e+02      2.500000e+02

        systolic BP    temperature           age        gender         height  \
count  1.015683e+06  321762.000000  1.461282e+06  1.461282e+06  455361.000000
mean   1.197054e+02      36.986995  6.535809e+01  1.554603e+00     169.170224
std    2.332119e+01       0.854016  1.663225e+01  4.970097e-01      14.552301
min    0.000000e+00      24.700000  1.803403e+01  1.000000e+00       0.000000
25%    1.030000e+02      36.444444  5.474257e+01  1.000000e+00     163.000000
50%    1.170000e+02      37.000000  6.738069e+01  2.000000e+00     170.000000
75%    1.340000e+02      37.500000  7.862746e+01  2.000000e+00     178.000000
max    4.110000e+02      42.222222  9.000000e+01  2.000000e+00     445.000000

                 pH        weight           day     mortality          hour
count  116414.000000  1.309930e+06  1.461282e+06  1.461282e+06  1.461282e+06
mean       7.368808  8.280987e+01  1.439831e+00  1.505267e-01  2.132638e+01
std        0.086337  2.575886e+01  4.963666e-01  3.575871e-01  1.420751e+01
min        6.800000  0.000000e+00  1.000000e+00  0.000000e+00  0.000000e+00
```

```
25%        7.320000  6.650000e+01  1.000000e+00  0.000000e+00  8.000000e+00
50%        7.380000  7.910000e+01  1.000000e+00  0.000000e+00  2.000000e+01
75%        7.420000  9.440000e+01  2.000000e+00  0.000000e+00  3.400000e+01
max        7.800000  9.312244e+02  2.000000e+00  1.000000e+00  4.700000e+01
```

The dataset consists of 21,139 unique ICU stays and 1,461,282 observations. All columns with the exception of 'hours', 'mortality' and 'day' have missing information. Looking at the maximum and minimum values it is possible to spot the presence of outliers (e.g. max glucose). Both missing data and outliers are very common in ICU databases and need to be taken into consideration before applying ML algorithms.

9.4 Variable Selection

In general, you should take into consideration the following criteria when deciding whether to include or exclude variables:

- adding more variables tends to decrease the sample size, because fewer patients are likely to have all of them collected at the same time;
- selecting a high number of variables might bias the dataset towards the selection of a specific group of patients whose characteristics required the measurement of those specific variables;
- variables should be independent with minimal correlation;
- the number of observations should be significantly higher than the number of variables, in order to avoid the curse of dimensionality.

Rejecting variables with an excessive number of missing values is usually a good rule of thumb. However, it might also lead to the reduction of predictive power and ability to detect significant differences. For these reasons, there should be a trade-off between the potential value of the variable in the model and the amount of data available. We already saw the amount of missing data for every column, but we still do not know how much information is missing at the patient level. In order to do so, we are going to aggregate data by ICU stay and look at the number of non-null values, using the 'groupby' function together with the 'mean' operator. This will give an indication of how many ICU stays have at least one observation for each variable.

Note that one patient might have multiple ICU stays. In this work, for the sake of simplicity, we will consider every ICU stay as an independent sample.

```
In [5]: print(data.groupby(['icustay']).mean().info(null_counts=1))
```

```
<class 'pandas.core.frame.DataFrame'>
Float64Index: 21139 entries, 200001.0 to 299995.0
Data columns (total 17 columns):
hours                  21139 non-null float64
diastolic BP           19154 non-null float64
glasgow coma scale     10993 non-null float64
glucose                18745 non-null float64
heart rate             19282 non-null float64
mean BP                19123 non-null float64
```

```
oxygen saturation       19305 non-null float64
respiratory rate        19367 non-null float64
systolic BP             19154 non-null float64
temperature             18440 non-null float64
age                     21139 non-null float64
gender                  21139 non-null float64
height                  5370 non-null float64
pH                      15489 non-null float64
weight                  18181 non-null float64
day                     21139 non-null float64
mortality               21139 non-null float64
dtypes: float64(17)
memory usage: 2.9 MB
None
```

Based on the previous information, some decisions are made:

- Height can be discarded due to the high amount of missing data;
- Weight and height are typically used in combination (body mass index), since individually they typically provide low predictive power. Therefore, weight was discarded;
- The other variables will be kept. Let us start analyzing time-variant variables and set aside age and gender for now:

```
In [6]: variables = ['diastolic BP', 'glasgow coma scale',
                     'glucose', 'heart rate', 'mean BP',
                     'oxygen saturation', 'respiratory rate', 'systolic BP',
                     'temperature', 'pH']
        variables_mort = variables.copy()
        variables_mort.append('mortality')
```

These decisions are specific for this case. Other criteria could have been used, for example, checking the correlation between all variables and excluding one variable out of every pair with high correlation in order to reduce redundancy.

9.5 Data Preprocessing

9.5.1 Outliers

9.5.1.1 Data Visualization

We already saw that outliers are present in the dataset, but we need to take a closer look at data before deciding how to handle them. Using the 'seaborn' library and the 'boxplot' function we can easily create one boxplot for every variable. Seaborn is a visualization library based on matplotlib that provides a high-level interface for drawing statistical graphics.

```
In [7]: import seaborn as sns

        fig = plt.figure(figsize=(10,10))
        count = 0
        for variable in variables:
            count += 1
            plt.subplot(4, 3, count)
            ax = sns.boxplot(y=variable, data=data)

        fig.tight_layout()
        plt.show()
```

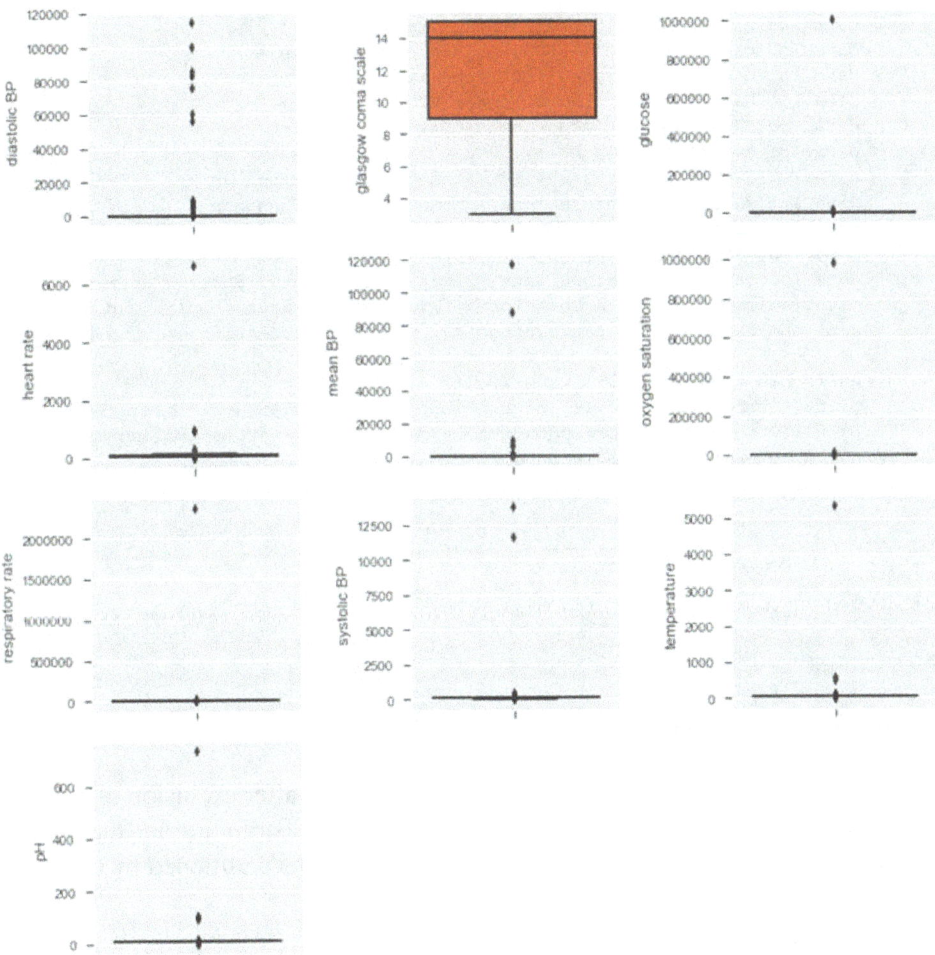

In some cases, the outliers are so deviant from the norm that it is not even possible to visualize the distribution of data (minimum, first quartile, median, third quartile, maximum) using boxplots. There are other plot types you can create to investigate the presence of outliers. Simply plotting all points using a scatter plot, or using violin plots are some of the options.

9.5.1.2 Exclusion

Ideally, we should keep extreme values related to the patients' poor health condition and exclude impossible values (such as negative temperature) and probable outliers (such as heart rate above 250 beats/min). In order to do so, values that fall outside boundaries defined by expert knowledge are excluded. This way, we avoid excluding extreme (but correct/possible) values.

```
In [8]: nulls_before = data.isnull().sum().sum()

        data.loc[data['diastolic BP']>300, 'diastolic BP'] = np.nan
        data.loc[data['glucose']>2000, 'glucose'] = np.nan
        data.loc[data['heart rate']>400, 'heart rate'] = np.nan
        data.loc[data['mean BP']>300, 'mean BP'] = np.nan
        data.loc[data['mean BP']<0, 'mean BP'] = np.nan
        data.loc[data['systolic BP']>10000,  'systolic BP'] = np.nan
        data.loc[data['temperature']>50, 'temperature'] = np.nan
        data.loc[data['temperature']<20, 'temperature'] = np.nan
        data.loc[data['pH']>7.8, 'pH'] = np.nan
        data.loc[data['pH']<6.8, 'pH'] = np.nan
        data.loc[data['respiratory rate']>300, 'respiratory rate'] = np.nan
        data.loc[data['oxygen saturation']>100, 'oxygen saturation'] = np.nan
        data.loc[data['oxygen saturation']<0, 'oxygen saturation'] = np.nan

        nulls_now = data.isnull().sum().sum()
        print('Number of observations removed: ' + str(nulls_now - nulls_before))
        print('Observations corresponding to outliers: ' + str(round((nulls_now -
        nulls_before)*100/data.shape[0],2)) + '%')
```

```
Number of observations removed: 7783
Observations corresponding to outliers: 0.53%
```

9.5.1.3 Data Visualization After Outliers Exclusion

The same code can be used to verify the data distribution after exclusion of outliers. The 'stripplot' function allows to visualize the underlying distribution and the number of observations. Setting x = 'mortality' shows the boxplots partitioned by outcome.

```
In [9]: fig = plt.figure(figsize=(10,10))
        count = 0
        for variable in variables:
            count += 1
            plt.subplot(4, 3, count)

            ax = sns.boxplot(x = 'mortality', y=variable, data=data)
            ax = sns.stripplot(x = 'mortality', y=variable, data=data, color="orange",
        jitter=0.2, size=0.5)

        fig.tight_layout()
        plt.show()
```

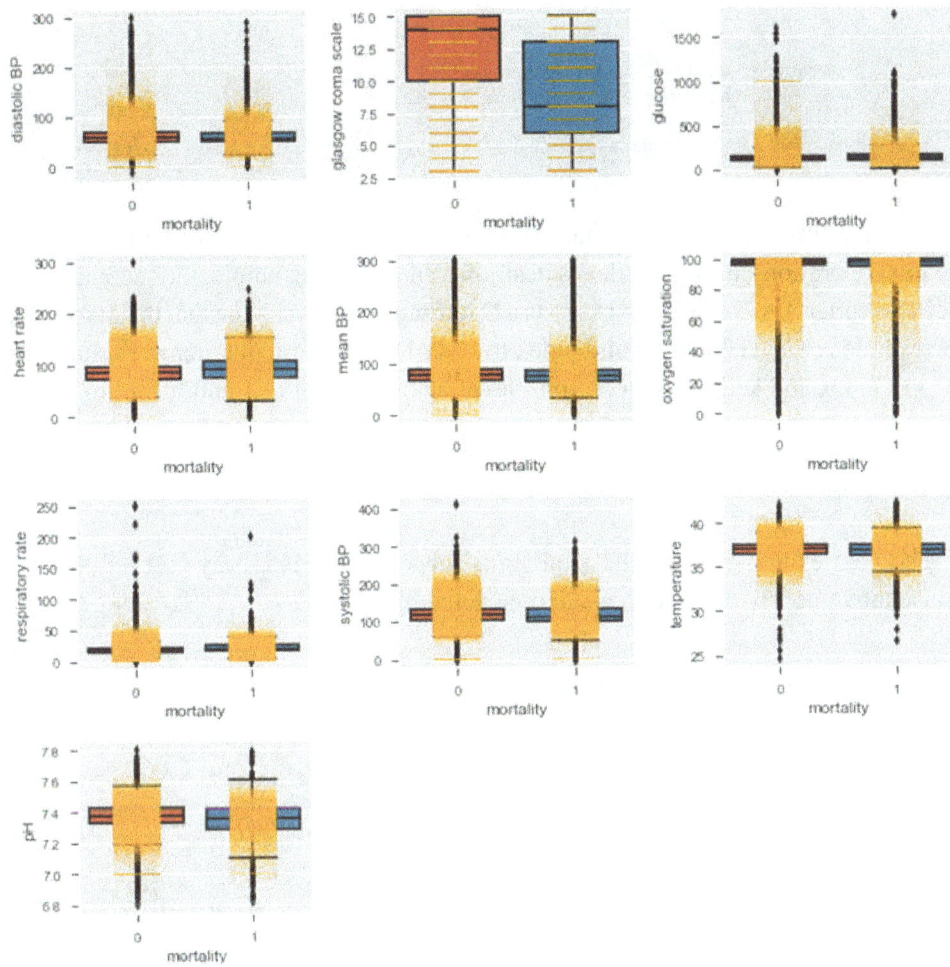

9.5.2 Aggregate Data by Hour

As mentioned before, the dataset contains information regarding the first 2 days in the ICU. Every observation is associated with a time stamp, indicating the number of hours elapsed between ICU admission and the time when the observation was collected (e.g., 0.63 h). To allow for ease of comparison, individual data is condensed into hourly observations by selecting the median value of the available observations within each hour. First, the 'floor' operator is applied in order to categorize the hours in 48 bins (hour 0, hour 1, ..., hour 47). Then, the 'groupby' function with the 'median' operator is applied in order to get the median heart rate for each hour of each ICU stay:

```
In [10]: data['hour'] = data['hours'].apply(np.floor)

         # data goes until h = 48, change 48 to 47
         data.loc[data['hour'] == 48, 'hour'] = 47

         data_median_hour = data.groupby(['icustay','hour'])[variables_mort].median()
```

The 'groupby' will create as many indexes as groups defined. In order to facilitate the next operations, a single index is desirable. In the next example, the second index (column 'hour') is excluded and kept as a DataFrame column. Note that the first index corresponds to level 0 and second index to level 1. Therefore, in order to exclude the second index and keep it as a column, 'level' should be set to 1 and 'drop' to False.

```
In [11]: data_median_hour = data_median_hour.reset_index(level=(1), drop = False)
```

The next example shows the vital signs for a specific ICU stay (ID = 200001). Consecutive hourly observations are connected by line.

```
In [12]: vitals = ['diastolic BP', 'heart rate', 'mean BP', 'oxygen saturation',
                   'respiratory rate', 'systolic BP','temperature']
         ICUstayID = 200001.0

         fig, ax = plt.subplots(figsize=(20,6))

         # scatter plot
         for col in vitals:
             ax.scatter(data_median_hour.loc[ICUstayID,'hour'],data_median_hour.loc[ICUstayID,col])
             plt.legend(loc=9, bbox_to_anchor=(0.5, -0.1), ncol=len(vitals), prop={'size': 14})
             plt.xticks(np.arange(0, 49, step=1))
             plt.xlabel('Hours since ICU admission')

         # connect consecutive points by line
         for col in vitals:
             ax.plot(data_median_hour.loc[ICUstayID,'hour'], data_median_hour.loc[ICUstayID,col])
```

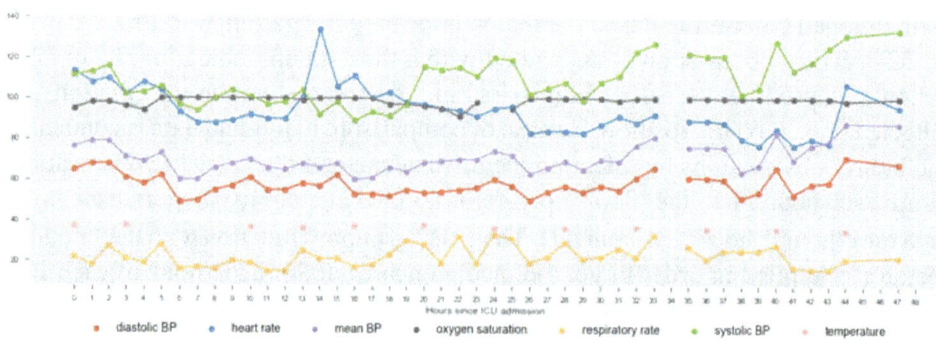

9.5.3 Select Minimum Number of Observations

We decided to keep all time-variant variables available. However, and as you can see in the previous example, since not all variables have a hourly sampling rate, a lot of information is missing (coded as NaN). In order to train ML algorithms it is important to decide how to handle the missing information. Two options are: to replace the missing information with some value or to exclude the missing information. In this work, we will avoid introducing bias resultant from replacing missing values with estimated values (which is not the same as saying that this is not a good option in some situations). Instead, we will focus on a complete case analysis, i.e., we will include in our analysis only those patients who have complete information.

Depending on how we will create the feature set, complete information can have different meanings. For example, if we want to use one observation for every hour, complete information is to have no missing data for every t = 0 to t = 47, which would lead to the exclusion of the majority of data. In order to reduce the size of the feature space, one common approach is to use only some portions of the time series. This is the strategy that will be followed in this work. Summary statistics, including the mean, maximum, minimum and standard deviation will be used to extract relevant information from the time series. In this case, it is important to define the minimum length of the time series before starting to select portions of it. One possible approach is to use all patients who have at least one observation per variable. Since, the summary statistics have little meaning if only one observation is available, a threshold of two observations is used.

In the following function, setting 'min_num_meas = 2' means that we are selecting ICU stays where each variable was recorded at least once at two different hours. Again, we are using the 'groupby' function to aggregate data by ICU stay, and the 'count' operator to count the number of observations for each variable. We then excluded ICU stays where some variable was recorded less than 2 times. Section 9.7 will show how to extract features from the time series.

```
In [13]: min_num_meas = 2


         def extr_min_num_meas(data_median_hour, min_num_meas):
             """ Select ICU stays where there are at least 'min_num_meas' observations
             and print the resulting DataFrame size"""
             data_count = data_median_hour.groupby(['icustay'])[variables_mort].count()

             for col in data_count:
                 data_count[col] = data_count[col].apply(lambda x: np.nan if x < min_num_meas
         else x)

             data_count = data_count.dropna(axis=0, how='any')
             print('Number of ICU stays: ' + str(data_count.shape[0]))
             print('Number of features: ' + str(data_count.shape[1]))
             unique_stays = data_count.index.unique()
```

```
        data_median_hour = data_median_hour.loc[unique_stays]

        return data_median_hour

    data_median_hour = extr_min_num_meas(data_median_hour, min_num_meas)
```

```
Number of ICU stays: 6931
Number of features: 11
```

It is always important to keep track of the size of data while making decisions about inclusion/exclusion criteria. We started with a database of around 60,000 ICU stays, imported a fraction of those that satisfied some criteria, in a total of 21,140 ICU stays, and are now looking at 6,931 ICU stays.

9.6 Data Analysis

9.6.1 Pairwise Ploting

One of the most used techniques in exploratory data analysis is the pairs plot (also called scatterplot). This technique allows to see both the distribution of single variables as well as relationships between every two variables. It is easily implemented in Python using the 'seaborn' library. The next example shows how to plot the pairwise relationships between variables and the histograms of single variables partitioned by outcome (survival vs non-survival). The argument 'vars' is used to indicate the set of variables to plot and 'hue' to indicate the use of different markers for each level of the 'hue' variable. A subset of data is used: 'dropna(axis = 0, how = 'any')' excludes all rows containing missing information.

```
In [14]: import seaborn as sns

         sns.set(style="ticks")
         g = sns.pairplot(data_median_hour[variables_mort].dropna(axis=0, how='any'), vars =
         variables, hue = 'mortality')

         # hide the upper triangle
         for i, j in zip(*np.triu_indices_from(g.axes, 1)):
             g.axes[i, j].set_visible(False)
         plt.show()

         # change back to our preferred style
         plt.style.use('ggplot')
```

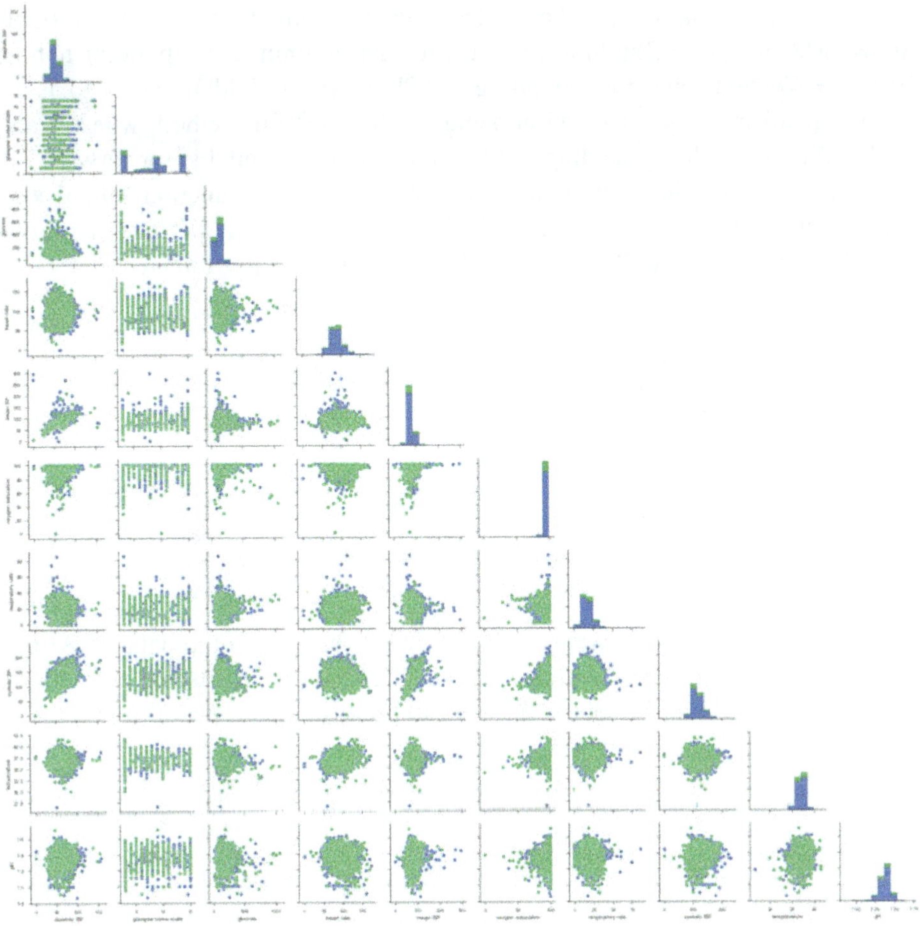

Unfortunately, this type of plot only allows to see relationships in a 2D space, which in most cases is not enough to find any patterns or trends. Nonetheless, it is still able to tell us important aspects of data; if not for showing promising directions for data analysis, to provide a means to check data's integrity. Things to highlight are:

- Hypoxic patients generally have lower SBPs;
- SBP correlates with MAP, which is a nice test of the data's integrity;
- Fever correlates with increasing tachycardia, also as expected.

9.6.2 *Time Series Ploting*

In order to investigate time trends, it is useful to visualize the mean HR partitioned by outcome from t = 0 to t = 47. In order to easily perform this task, the DataFrame needs to be restructured.

The next function takes as input a pandas DataFrame and the name of the variable and transposes/pivots the DataFrame in order to have columns corresponding to time (t = 0 to t = 47) and rows corresponding to ICU stays. If 'filldata' is set to 1, the function will fill missing information using the forward fill method, where NaNs are replaced by the value preceding it. In case no value is available for forward fill, NaNs are replaced by the next value in the time series. The function 'fillna' with the method argument set to 'ffill' and 'bfill', allows us to easily perform these two actions. If 'filldata' is set to 0 no missing data imputation is performed.

```
In [15]: def timeseries_data(data_median_hour, variable, filldata = 1):
             """Return matrix of time series data for clustering,
             with rows corresponding to unique observations (ICU stays) and
             columns corresponding to time since ICU admission"""
             data4clustering = data_median_hour.pivot(columns='hour', values=variable)
             if filldata == 1:
                 # first forward fill
                 data4clustering = data4clustering.fillna(method='ffill', axis=1)
                 # next backward fill
                 data4clustering = data4clustering.fillna(method='bfill', axis=1)
                 data4clustering = data4clustering.dropna(axis=0, how='all')
             return data4clustering
```

The next script plots the average HR for every variable in the dataset. At this point, 'filldata' is set to 0. In the section named Time Series Clustering of Part II of this tutorial, 'filldata' will be set to 1 in order to perform clustering of time series.

```
In [16]: fig = plt.figure(figsize=(10,10))
         count = 0
         for variable in variables:
             count += 1
             data4clustering = timeseries_data(data_median_hour, variable, filldata = 0)
             print('Plotting ' + str(data4clustering.count().sum()) + ' observations from ' +
         str(data4clustering.shape[0]) + ' ICU stays' + ' - ' + variable)
             class1 = data4clustering.loc[data[data['mortality']==1].index.unique()].mean()
             class0 = data4clustering.loc[data[data['mortality']==0].index.unique()].mean()
             plt.subplot(4, 3, count)
             plt.plot(class1)
             plt.plot(class0)
             plt.xlabel('Hours since ICU admission')
             plt.ylabel('Mean ' + variable)

         fig.tight_layout()
         plt.legend(['Non-survivors', 'Survivors'])
         plt.show()
```

```
Plotting 308913 observations from 6931 ICU stays - diastolic BP
Plotting 107073 observations from 6931 ICU stays - glasgow coma scale
Plotting 99885 observations from 6931 ICU stays - glucose
Plotting 310930 observations from 6931 ICU stays - heart rate
Plotting 306827 observations from 6931 ICU stays - mean BP
Plotting 302563 observations from 6931 ICU stays - oxygen saturation
Plotting 305363 observations from 6931 ICU stays - respiratory rate
Plotting 308942 observations from 6931 ICU stays - systolic BP
Plotting 138124 observations from 6931 ICU stays - temperature
Plotting 60375 observations from 6931 ICU stays - pH
```

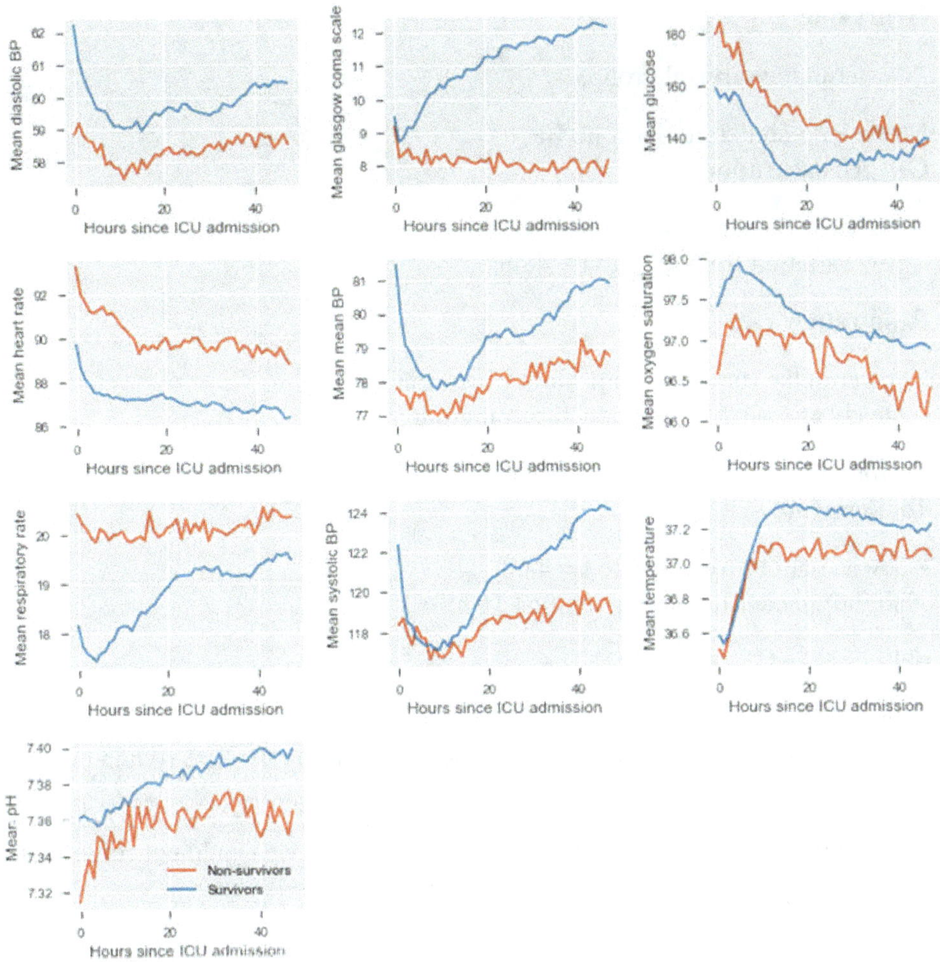

The physiological deterioration or improvement over time is very different between survivors and non-survivors. While using the pairwise plot we could not see any differences between the groups, this type of plot reveals very clear differences. Several observations can be made:

- **Diastolic BP**
  - higher in the survival group;
  - rapidly decreasing during the first 10 h, especially in the survival group, and increasing at a lower rate thereafter;
- **Glasgow coma scale**
  - higher in the survival group, increasing over time;
  - steady around 8 in the non-survival group;
  - similar between both groups at admission, but diverging thereafter;
- **Glucose**
  - decreasing over time in both groups;

- **Heart rate**
  - lower in the survival group;
- **Mean BP** - similar to diastolic BP;
- **Oxygen saturation**
  - higher in the survival group;
  - low variation from t = 0 to t = 48 h;
- **Respiratory rate**
  - lower in the survival group, slowly increasing over time;
  - steady around 20 in the non-survival group;
- **Systolic BP**—similar to diastolic and mean BP;
- **Temperature**
  - low variation from t = 0 to t = 48 h;
  - slightly increasing during the first 10 h;
- **pH**
  - Increasing over time in both groups;
  - pH < 7.35 (associated with metabolic acidosis) during the first 10 h in the non-survival group.

Most of these graphs have fairly interesting trends, but we would not consider the oxygen saturation or temperature graphs to be clinically relevant.

9.7 Feature Construction

The next step before ML is to extract relevant features from the time series. As already mentioned, the complete time series could be used for ML, however, missing information would have to be filled or excluded. Also, using the complete time series would result in $48\text{h} \times 11\text{variables} = 528$ features, which would make the models difficult to interpret and could lead to overfitting. There is a simpler solution, which is to use only a portion of the information available, ideally the most relevant information for the prediction task.

Feature construction addresses the problem of finding the transformation of variables containing the greatest amount of useful information. In this chapter, simple operations will be used to construct/extract important features from the time series:

- Maximum
- Minimum
- Standard deviation
- Mean

Other summary statistics or time-series snapshots could have been used, for example, the median, time elapsed between maximum and minimum, time elapsed between baseline and maximum, difference between baseline and minimum, and others. Alternatively, other techniques can be used for dimensionality reduction, such as principal component analysis (PCA) and autoencoders described in the previous Chapter.

The maximum, minimum, standard deviation and mean summarize the worst, best, variation and average patient' condition from t = 0 to t = 47h. In the proposed exercises you will do this for each day separately, which will increase the dataset dimensionality but hopefully will allow the extraction of more useful information. Using the 'groupby' function to aggregate data by ICU stay, together with the 'max', 'min', 'std' and 'mean' operators, these features can be easily extracted:

```
In [17]: def feat_transf(data):
             data_max = data.groupby(['icustay'])[variables].max()
             data_max.columns = ['max ' + str(col) for col in data_max.columns]

             data_min = data.groupby(['icustay'])[variables].min()
             data_min.columns = ['min ' + str(col) for col in data_min.columns]

             data_sd = data.groupby(['icustay'])[variables].std()
             data_sd.columns = ['sd ' + str(col) for col in data_sd.columns]

             data_mean = data.groupby(['icustay'])[variables].mean()
             data_mean.columns = ['mean ' + str(col) for col in data_mean.columns]

             data_agg = pd.concat([data_min,data_max,data_sd,data_mean],axis=1)

             return data_agg

         data_transf = feat_transf(data_median_hour).dropna(axis=0)

         print('Extracted features: ')
         display.display(data_transf.columns)
         print('')
         print('Number of ICU stays: ' + str(data_transf.shape[0]))
         print('Number of features: ' + str(data_transf.shape[1]))
```

```
Extracted features:
```

```
Index(['min diastolic BP', 'min glasgow coma scale', 'min glucose',
       'min heart rate', 'min mean BP', 'min oxygen saturation',
       'min respiratory rate', 'min systolic BP', 'min temperature', 'min pH',
       'max diastolic BP', 'max glasgow coma scale', 'max glucose',
       'max heart rate', 'max mean BP', 'max oxygen saturation',
       'max respiratory rate', 'max systolic BP', 'max temperature', 'max pH',
       'sd diastolic BP', 'sd glasgow coma scale', 'sd glucose',
       'sd heart rate', 'sd mean BP', 'sd oxygen saturation',
       'sd respiratory rate', 'sd systolic BP', 'sd temperature', 'sd pH',
       'mean diastolic BP', 'mean glasgow coma scale', 'mean glucose',
       'mean heart rate', 'mean mean BP', 'mean oxygen saturation',
       'mean respiratory rate', 'mean systolic BP', 'mean temperature',
       'mean pH'],
      dtype='object')
```

```
Number of ICU stays: 6931
Number of features: 40
```

A DataFrame containing one row per ICU stay was obtained, where each column corresponds to one feature. We are one step closer to building the models. Next, we are going to add the time invariant information—age and gender—to the dataset.

```
In [18]: mortality = data.loc[data_transf.index]['mortality'].groupby(['icustay']).mean()
         age = data.loc[data_transf.index]['age'].groupby(['icustay']).mean()
         gender = data.loc[data_transf.index]['gender'].groupby(['icustay']).mean()

         data_transf_inv = pd.concat([data_transf, age, gender, mortality],
         axis=1).dropna(axis=0)
         print('Number of ICU stays: ' + str(data_transf_inv.shape[0]))
         print('Number of features: ' + str(data_transf_inv.shape[1]))
```

```
Number of ICU stays: 6931
Number of features: 43
```

9.8 Data Partitioning

In order to assess the performance of the models, data can be divided into training, test and validation sets as exemplified in Fig. 9.1. This is known as the holdout validation method. The training set is used to train/build the learning algorithm; the validation (or development) set is used to tune parameters, select features, and make other decisions regarding the learning algorithm and the test set is used to evaluate the performance of the algorithm, but not to make any decisions regarding the learning algorithm architecture or parameters.

For simplicity, data is divided into two sets, one for training and another for testing. Later, when performing feature selection, the training set will be divided into two sets, for training and validation.

Scikit-learn is the essential machine learning package in Python. It provides simple and efficient tools for data mining and data analysis. The next example shows how to use the 'train_test_split' function from 'sklearn' library to randomly assign observations to each set. The size of the sets can be controlled using the 'test_size' parameter, which defines the size of the test set and which in this case is set to 20%. When using the 'train_test_split' function, it is important to set the 'random_state' parameter so that later the same results can be reproduced.

```
In [23]: from sklearn.cross_validation import train_test_split

         # set the % of observations in the test set
         test_size = 0.2

         # Divide the data intro training and test sets
         X_train, X_test, y_train, y_test = train_test_split(data_transf_inv,
         data_transf_inv[['mortality']], test_size = test_size, random_state = 10)
```

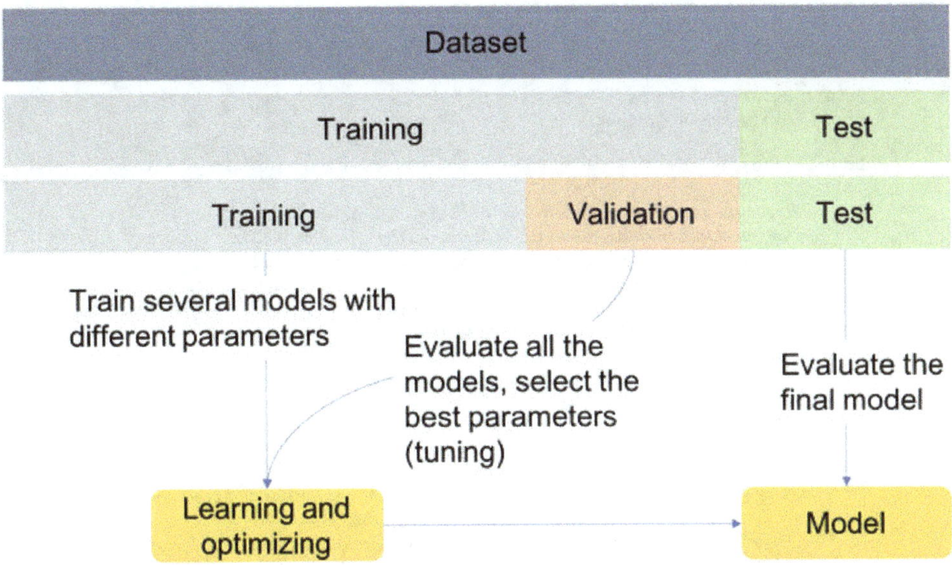

Fig. 9.1 Illustrative scheme of the holdout validation method

It is useful to create a function that prints the size of data in each set:

```
In [24]: def print_size(y_train, y_test):
             print(str(len(y_train[y_train['mortality']==1])) + '(' +
         str(round(len(y_train[y_train['mortality']==1])/len(y_train)*100,1)) + '%)' + ' non-
         survivors in training set')
             print(str(len(y_train[y_train['mortality']==0])) + '(' +
         str(round(len(y_train[y_train['mortality']==0])/len(y_train)*100,1)) + '%)' + '
         survivors in training set')
             print(str(len(y_test[y_test['mortality']==1])) + '(' +
         str(round(len(y_test[y_test['mortality']==1])/len(y_test)*100,1)) + '%)' + ' non-
         survivors in test set')
             print(str(len(y_test[y_test['mortality']==0])) + '(' +
         str(round(len(y_test[y_test['mortality']==0])/len(y_test)*100,1)) + '%)' + ' survivors
         in test set')
```

In cases where the data is highly imbalanced, it might be a good option to force an oversampling of the minority class, or an undersampling of the majority class so that the model is not biased towards the majority class. This should be performed on the training set, whereas the test set should maintain the class imbalance found on the original data, so that when evaluating the final model a true representation of data is used.

For the purpose of facilitating clustering interpretability, undersampling is used. However, as a general rule of thumb, and unless the dataset contains a huge number of observations, oversampling is preferred over undersampling because it allows keeping all the information in the training set. In any case, selecting learning algorithms that account for class imbalance might be a better choice.

The next example shows how to undersample the majority class, given a desired size of the minority class, controlled by the parameter 'perc_class1'. If 'perc_class1'>0, undersampling is performed in order to have a balanced training set. If 'perc_class1' = 0, no balancing is performed.

```
In [25]: # set the % of class 1 samples to be present in the training set.
         perc_class1 = 0.4

         print('Before balancing')
         print_size(y_train, y_test)

         if perc_class1 > 0:

             # Find the indices of class 0 and class 1 samples
             class0_indices = y_train[y_train['mortality'] == 0].index
             class1_indices = y_train[y_train['mortality'] == 1].index

             # Calculate the number of samples for the majority class (survivors)
             class0_size = round(np.int((len(y_train[y_train['mortality'] == 1])*(1 -
         perc_class1)) / perc_class1),0)

             # Set the random seed generator for reproducibility
             np.random.seed(10)

             # Random sample majority class indices
             random_indices = np.random.choice(class0_indices, class0_size, replace=False)

             # Concat class 0 with class 1 indices
             X_train = pd.concat([X_train.loc[random_indices],X_train.loc[class1_indices]])
             y_train = pd.concat([y_train.loc[random_indices],y_train.loc[class1_indices]])

             print('After balancing')
             print_size(y_train, y_test)

         # Exclude output from input data
         X_train = X_train.drop(columns = 'mortality')
         X_test = X_test.drop(columns = 'mortality')
```

```
Before balancing
941(17.0%) non--survivors in training set
4603(83.0%) survivors in training set
246(17.7%) non--survivors in test set
1141(82.3%) survivors in test set
After balancing
941(40.0%) non--survivors in training set
1411(60.0%) survivors in training set
246(17.7%) non--survivors in test set
1141(82.3%) survivors in test set
```

In the following "Part 2 - Unsupervised Learning with Clustering", clustering will be used to identify patterns in the dataset.

Acknowledgements This work was supported by the Portuguese Foundation for Science and Technology, through IDMEC, under LAETA, project UID/EMS/50022/2019 and LISBOA-01-0145-FEDER-031474 supported by Programa Operacional Regional de Lisboa by FEDER and FCT.

10

Machine Learning for Phenotyping: Clustering and Unsupervised Learning

Cátia M. Salgado and Susana M. Vieira

Abstract Machine Learning for Phenotyping is composed of three chapters and aims to introduce clinicians to machine learning (ML). It provides a guideline through the basic concepts underlying machine learning and the tools needed to easily implement it using the Python programming language and Jupyter notebook documents. It is divided into three main parts: part 1—data preparation and analysis; part 2—unsupervised learning for clustering and part 3—supervised learning for classification.

Keywords Machine learning · Phenotyping · Data preparation · Data analysis · Unsupervised learning · Clustering · Supervised learning · Classification · Clinical informatics

10.1 Clustering

Clustering is a learning task that aims to decompose a given set of observations into subgroups (clusters) based on data similarity, such that observations in the same cluster are more closely related to each other than observations in different clusters. It is an unsupervised learning task, since it identifies structures in unlabeled datasets, and a classification task, since it can give a label to observations according to the cluster they are assigned to. For a more detailed description of supervised and unsupervised learning please refer to the previous chapter.

This work focuses on the following questions:

- Can we identify distinct patterns even if the class labels are not provided?
- How are the different patterns represented across different outcomes?

In order to address these questions, we will start by providing a description of the basic concepts underlying k-means clustering, which is the most well known and simple clustering algorithm. We will show how the algorithm works using 2D data

C. M. Salgado (✉) · S. M. Vieira
IDMEC, Instituto Superior Técnico, Universidade de Lisboa, Av. Rovisco Pais, Lisboa, Portugal
e-mail: catia.salgado@tecnico.ulisboa.pt

as an example, perform clustering of time series and use the information gained with clustering to train predictive models. The k-means clustering algorithm is described next.

10.1.1 K-means Clustering Algorithm

Consider a (training) dataset composed of N observations:

$$x_1, x_2, ..., x_N$$

Initialize K centroids $\mu_1, \mu_2, ..., \mu_K$ randomly.
Repeat until convergence:

1. Cluster assignment
   Assign each x_i to the nearest cluster. For every i do:

$$\underset{j}{argmin} \left\| x_i - \mu_j \right\|^2,$$

   where $j = 1, 2, ..., K$.
2. Cluster updating
   Update the cluster centroids μ_j. For every j do:

$$\mu_j = \frac{1}{N_j} \left[x_1^j + x_2^j + ... + x_{N_j}^j \right],$$

   where N_j is the number of observations assigned to cluster $j, k = 1, 2, ..., N_j$, and x_k^j represents observation k assigned to cluster j. Each new centroid corresponds to the mean of the observations assigned in the previous step.

10.1.2 Exemplification with 2D Data

Although pairwise plots did not reveal any interesting patterns, some clusters might have emerged after the data were transformed. You can re-run the code for pairwise plots between transformed features, but note that it will be time consuming due to the high dimensionality of the dataset. Features 'max mean BP' and 'mean heart rate' were chosen for illustrative purposes. The dataset is plotted below:

```
In [26]: x1 = 'max mean BP'
         x2 = 'mean heart rate'
         sns.lmplot(x1, x2, data_transf_inv, hue="mortality", fit_reg=False);
```

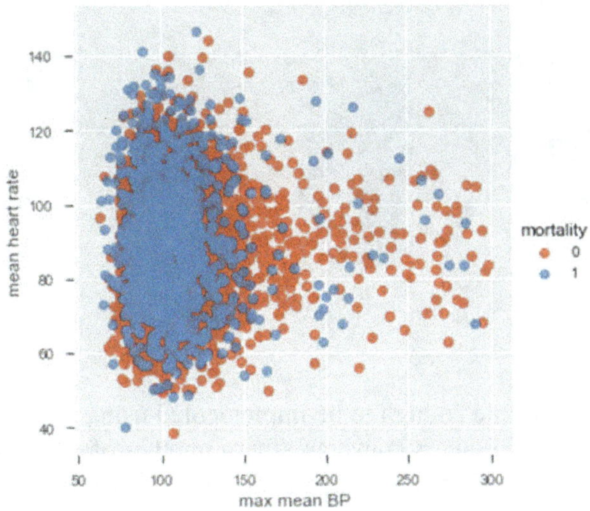

The number of clusters (K) must be provided before running k-means. It is not easy to guess the number of clusters just by looking at the previous plot, but for the purpose of understanding how the algorithm works 3 clusters are used. As usual, the 'random_state' parameter is predefined. Note that it does not matter which value is defined; the important thing is that this way we guarantee that when using the predefined value we will always get the same results.

The next example shows how to perform k-means using 'sklearn'.

```
In [27]: from sklearn.cluster import KMeans

         # set the number of clusters
         K = 3

         # input data to fit K-means
         X = pd.DataFrame.as_matrix(data_transf_inv[[x1,x2]])

         # fit kmeans
         kmeans = KMeans(n_clusters=K, random_state=0).fit(data_transf_inv[[x1,x2]])
```

The attribute 'labels_' gives the labels that indicate to which cluster each observation belongs, and 'cluster_centers_' gives the coordinates of cluster centers representing the mean of all observations in the cluster. Using these two attributes it is possible to plot the cluster centers and the data in each cluster using different colors to distinguish the clusters:

```
In [28]: classes = kmeans.labels_
         centroids = kmeans.cluster_centers_

         # define a colormap
         colormap = plt.get_cmap('tab20')
         for c in range(K):
             centroids[c] = np.mean(X[classes == c], 0)
             plt.scatter(x = X[classes == c,0], y = X[classes == c,1], alpha = 0.4, c =
         colormap(c))
             plt.scatter(x = centroids[c,0], y = centroids[c,1], c = 'black', marker='x')

         plt.xlabel(x1)
         plt.ylabel(x2)
         display.clear_output(wait=True)
```

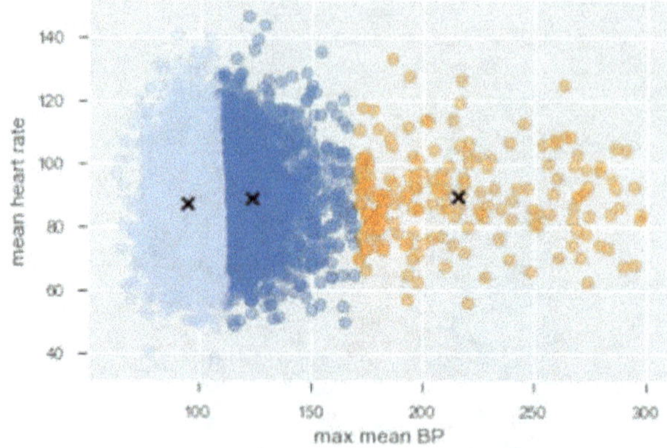

The algorithm is simple enough to be implemented using a few lines of code. If you want to see how the centers converge after a number of iterations, you can use the code below, which is an implementation of the k-means clustering algorithm step by step.

```
In [29]: # The following code was adapted from http://jonchar.net/notebooks/k-means/
         import time
         from IPython import display

         K = 3

         def initialize_clusters(points, k):
             """Initializes clusters as k randomly selected coordinates."""
             return points[np.random.randint(points.shape[0], size=k)]

         def get_distances(centroid, points):
             """Returns the distance between centroids and observations."""
             return np.linalg.norm(points - centroid, axis=1)

         # Initialize centroids
         centroids = initialize_clusters(X, K)
         centroids_old = np.zeros([K, X.shape[1]], dtype=np.float64)

         # Initialize the vectors in which the assigned classes
         # of each observation will be stored and the
         # calculated distances from each centroid
         classes = np.zeros(X.shape[0], dtype=np.float64)
         distances = np.zeros([X.shape[0], K], dtype=np.float64)

         # Loop until convergence of centroids
         error = 1
         while error>0:

             # Assign all observations to the nearest centroid
             for i, c in enumerate(centroids):
                 distances[:, i] = get_distances(c, X)

             # Determine class membership of each observation
             # by picking the closest centroid
             classes = np.argmin(distances, axis=1)

             # Update centroid location using the newly
             # assigned observations classes
             # Change to median in order to have k-medoids
             for c in range(K):
                 centroids[c] = np.mean(X[classes == c], 0)
                 plt.scatter(x = X[classes == c,0], y = X[classes == c,1], alpha = 0.4, c =
         colormap(c))
                 plt.scatter(x = centroids[c,0], y = centroids[c,1], c = 'black', marker='x')
```

```
        error = sum(get_distances(centroids, centroids_old))
        centroids_old = centroids.copy()

        #pl.text(max1, min2, str(error))
        plt.xlabel(x1)
        plt.ylabel(x2)
        display.clear_output(wait=True)
        display.display(plt.gcf())
        time.sleep(0.01)
        plt.gcf().clear()
```

Please refer to the online material in order to visualize the plot. It shows the position of the cluster centers at each iteration, until convergence to the final centroids. The trajectory of the centers depends on the cluster initialization; because the initialization is random, the centers might not always converge to the same position.

10.1.3 Time Series Clustering

Time series analysis revealed distinct and interesting patterns across survivors and non-survivors. Next, k-means clustering is used to investigate patterns in time series. The goal is to stratify patients according to their evolution in the ICU, from admission to t = 48 h, for every variable separately. Note that at this point we are back to working with time series information instead of constructed features.

For this particular task and type of algorithm, it is important to normalize data for each patient separately. This will allow a comparison between time trends rather than a comparison between the magnitude of observations. In particular, if the data is normalized individually for each patient, clustering will tend to group together patients that (for example) started with the lowest values and ended up with the highest values, whereas if the data is not normalized, the same patients might end up in different clusters because of the magnitude of the signal, even though the trend is similar.

Missing data is filled forward, i.e., missing values are replaced with the value preceding it (the last known value at any point in time). If there is no information preceding a missing value, these are replaced by the following values.

```
In [30]: # Now we are going to pivot the table in order to have rows corresponding to unique
         # ICU stays and columns corresponding to hour since admission. This will be used for
         clustering

         def clustering(variable, ids_clustering, K, *args):
             """Return data for clustering, labels attributted to training observations and
             if *args is provided return labels attributted to test observations"""

             data4clustering = timeseries_data(data_median_hour, variable, filldata = 1)

             # data for clustering is normalized by patient
             # since the data is normalized by patient we can normalize training and test data
         together
             for index, row in data4clustering.iterrows():
                 maxx = data4clustering.loc[index].max()
                 minn = data4clustering.loc[index].min()
                 data4clustering.loc[index] = (data4clustering.loc[index] - minn) / (maxx-minn)
```

```
    # select data for creating the clusters
    data4clustering_train = data4clustering.loc[ids_clustering].dropna(axis=0)
    print('Using ' + str(data4clustering_train.shape[0]) + ' ICU stays for creating the
clusters')

    # create the clusters
    kmeans = KMeans(n_clusters = K, random_state = 2).fit(data4clustering_train)
    centers = kmeans.cluster_centers_
    labels = kmeans.labels_

    # test the clusters if test data is provided
    labels_test = []
    for arg in args:
        data4clustering_test = data4clustering.loc[arg].set_index(arg).dropna(axis=0)
        labels_test = kmeans.predict(data4clustering_test)
        labels_test = pd.DataFrame(labels_test).set_index(data4clustering_test.index)
        print('Using ' + str(data4clustering_test.shape[0]) + ' ICU stays for cluster
assignment')

    print(str(K) + ' clusters')
    cluster=0
    d = {}
    mortality_cluster = {}

    colormap1 = plt.get_cmap('jet')
    colors = colormap1(np.linspace(0,1,K))

    fig1 = plt.figure(1, figsize=(15,4))
    fig2 = plt.figure(2, figsize=(15,3))

    for center in centers:
        ax1 = fig1.add_subplot(1,2,1)
        ax1.plot(center, color = colors[cluster])

        ax2 = fig2.add_subplot(1,K,cluster+1)
        data_cluster =  data4clustering_train.iloc[labels==cluster]
        ax2.plot(data_cluster.transpose(),  alpha = 0.1, color = 'silver')
        ax2.plot(center, color = colors[cluster])
        ax2.set_xlabel('Hours since admission')
        if cluster == 0:
            ax2.set_ylabel('Normalized ' + variable)
        ax2.set_ylim((0, 1))
        cluster += 1
        data_cluster_mort =
data['mortality'].loc[data_cluster.index].groupby(['icustay']).mean()
        print('Cluster ' + str(cluster) + ': ' + str(data_cluster.shape[0]) + '
observations')
        mortality_cluster[cluster] = sum(data_cluster_mort)/len(data_cluster_mort)*100
        d[cluster] = str(cluster)

    labels = pd.DataFrame(labels).set_index(data4clustering_train.index)

    ax1.legend(d)
    ax1.set_xlabel('Hours since ICU admission')
    ax1.set_ylabel('Normalized ' + variable)
    ax1.set_ylim((0, 1))

    ax3 = fig1.add_subplot(1,2,2)
    x, y = zip(*mortality_cluster.items())
    ax3.bar(x, y, color=colors)
    ax3.set_xlabel('Cluster')
    ax3.set_ylabel('Non-survivors (%)')
    ax3.set_xticks(np.arange(1, K+1, step=1))

    plt.show()

    if args:
        return data4clustering, labels, labels_test
    else:
        return data4clustering, labels
```

10.1.3.1 Visual Inspection of the Best Number of Clusters for Each Variable

In the next example, k-means clustering is performed for glasgow coma scale (GCS), for a varying number of clusters (K). Only the training data is used to identify the clusters. The figures show, by order of appearance: cluster centers, percentage of non-survivors in each cluster, and cluster centers and training data in each cluster.

```
In [31]: variable = 'glasgow coma scale'
         clusters = range(2, 6)

         ids_clustering = X_train.index.unique()
         for K in clusters:
             data4clustering, cluster_labels = clustering(variable, ids_clustering, K)
```

```
Using 2110 ICU stays for creating the clusters
2 clusters
Cluster 1: 1215 observations
Cluster 2: 895 observations
```

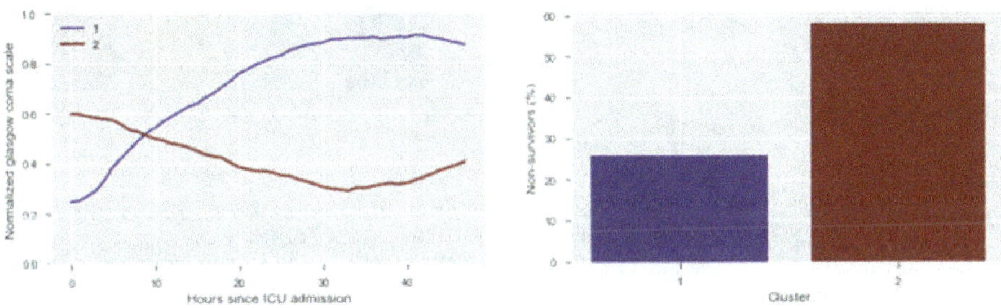

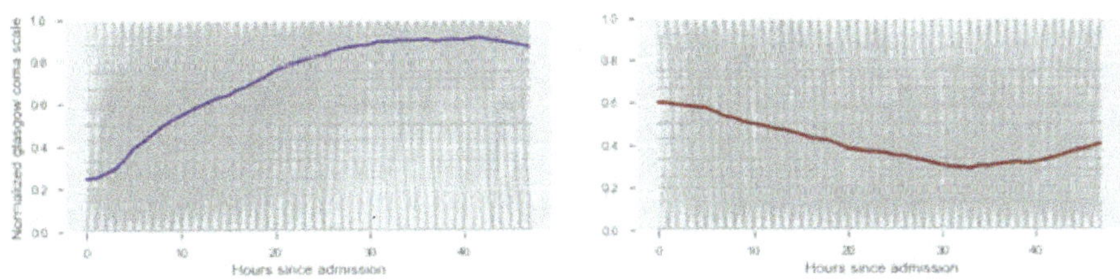


```
Using 2110 ICU stays for creating the clusters
3 clusters
Cluster 1: 806 observations
Cluster 2: 631 observations
Cluster 3: 673 observations
```

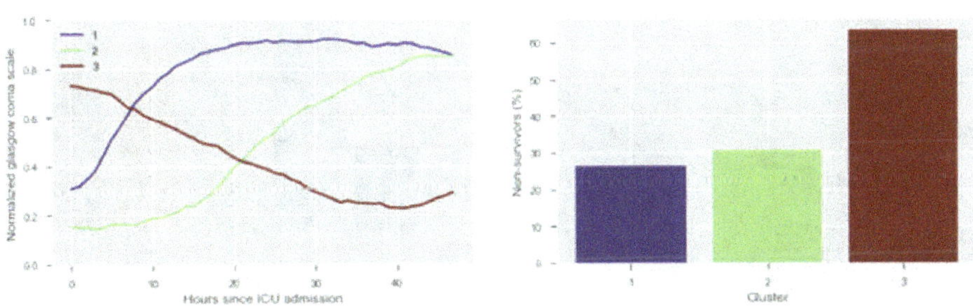

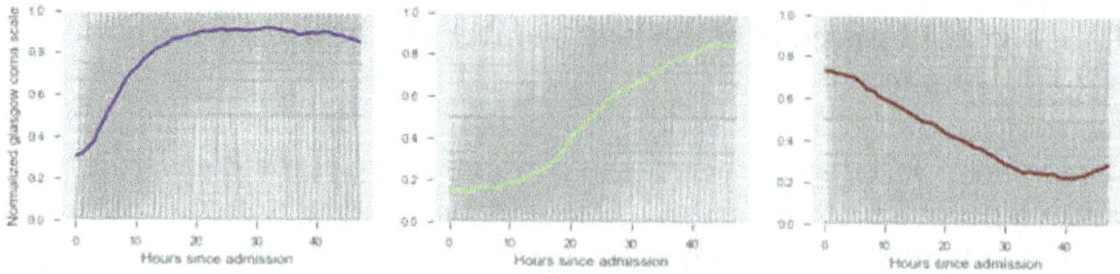


```
Using 2110 ICU stays for creating the clusters
4 clusters
Cluster 1: 579 observations
Cluster 2: 578 observations
Cluster 3: 453 observations
Cluster 4: 500 observations
```

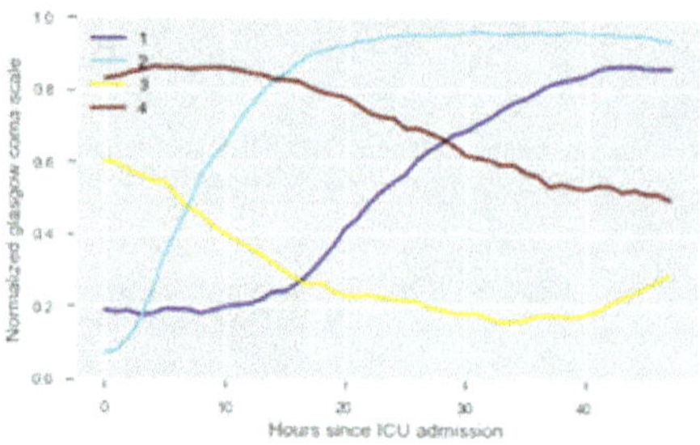

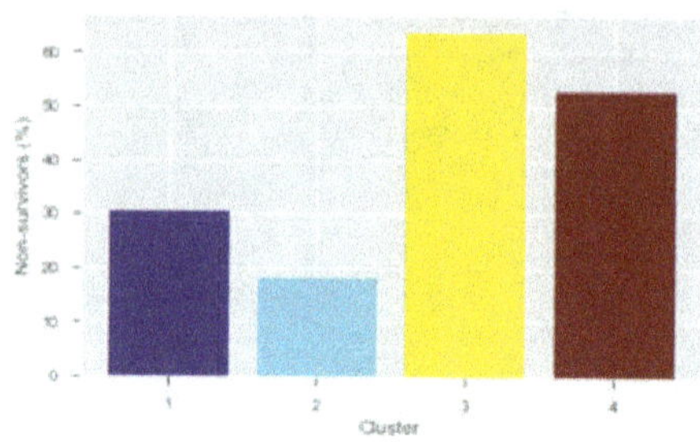

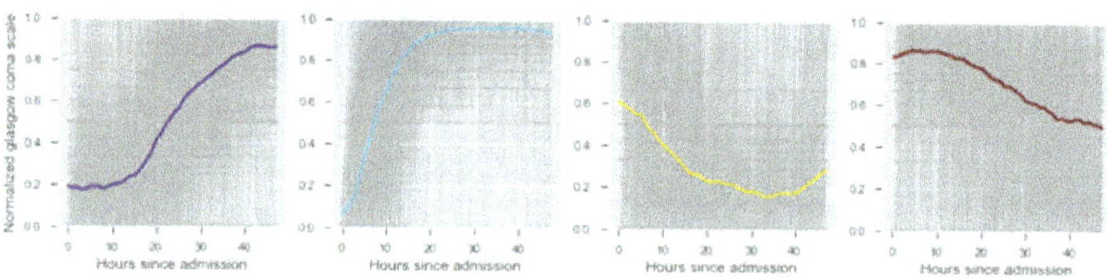


```
Using 2110 ICU stays for creating the clusters
5 clusters
Cluster 1: 471 observations
Cluster 2: 328 observations
Cluster 3: 514 observations
Cluster 4: 464 observations
Cluster 5: 333 observations
```

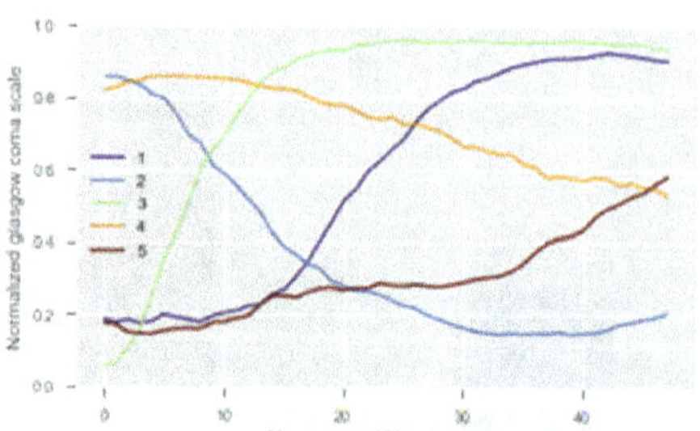

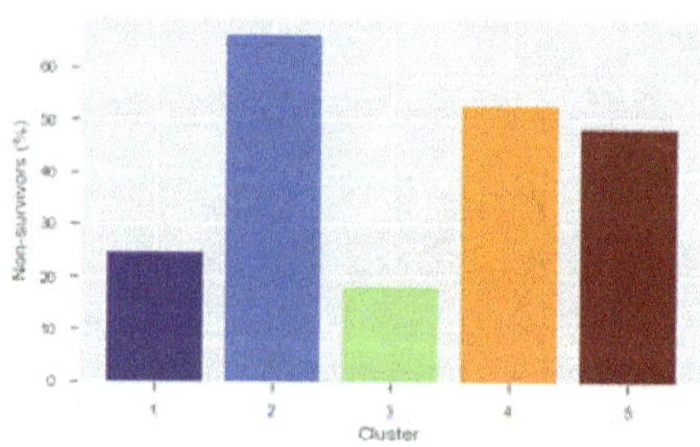

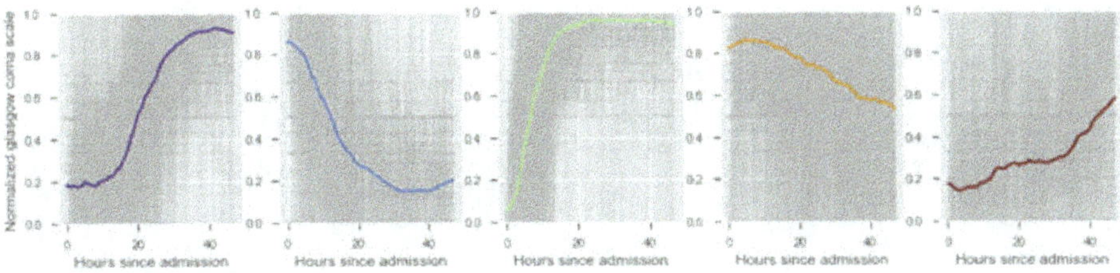

The goal of plotting cluster centers, mortality distribution and data in each cluster is to visually inspect the quality of the clusters. Another option would be to use quantitative methods, typically known as cluster validity indices, that automatically give the "best" number of clusters according to some criteria (e.g., cluster compacteness, cluster separation). Some interesting findings are:

- $K = 2$
  - shows two very distinct patterns, similar to what was found by partitioning by mortality;
  - but, we probably want more stratification.
- $K = 3$
  - 2 groups where GCS is improving with time;
  - 1 group where GCS is deteriorating;
  - yes, this is reflected in terms of our ground truth labels, even though we did not provide that information to the clustering. Mortality$>$ 60% in one cluster versus 30% and 28% in the other two clusters.
- $K = 4$
  - one more "bad" cluster appears.
- $K = 5$
  - Clusters 2 and 4 have similar patterns and similar mortality distribution. GCS is improving with time;
  - Clusters 3 and 5 have similar mortality distribution. GCS is slowly increasing or decreasing with time;
  - Cluster 1 is the "worst" cluster. Mortality is close to 70%.

In summary, every K from 2 to 5 gives an interesting view of the evolution of GCS and its relation with mortality. For the sake of simplicity, this analysis is only shown for GCS. You can investigate on your own the cluster tendency for other variables and decide what is a good number of clusters for all of them. For now, the following K is used for each variable:

```
In [32]: # create a dictionary of selected K for each variable
         Ks = dict([('diastolic BP', 4),
                    ('glasgow coma scale', 4),
                    ('glucose', 5),
                    ('heart rate', 5),
                    ('mean BP', 5),
                    ('oxygen saturation', 3),
```

```
                    ('respiratory rate', 5),
                    ('systolic BP', 4),
                    ('temperature', 4),
                    ('pH', 4),
                   ])
```

10.1.3.2 Training and Testing

In this work, cluster labels are used to add another layer of information to the machine learning models. During the training phase, clustering is performed on the time series from the training set. Cluster centers are created and training observations are assigned to each cluster. During the test phase, test observations are assigned to one of the clusters defined in the training phase. Each observation is assigned to the most similar cluster, i.e., to the cluster whose center is at a smaller distance. These observations are not used to identify clusters centers.

The next example trains/creates and tests/assigns clusters using the 'clustering' function previously defined. Cluster labels are stored in 'cluster_labels_train' and 'cluster_labels_test'.

```
In [33]: id_train = X_train.index.unique()
         id_test = X_test.index.unique()
         cluster_labels_train = pd.DataFrame()
         cluster_labels_test = pd.DataFrame()

         for feature in variables:
             print(feature)
             K = Ks[feature]
             data4clustering, labels_train, labels_test = clustering(feature, id_train, K,
         id_test)

             labels_test.columns=['CL ' + feature]
             labels_train.columns=['CL ' + feature]

             cluster_labels_train = pd.concat([cluster_labels_train, labels_train],
         axis=1).dropna(axis=0)
             cluster_labels_test = pd.concat([cluster_labels_test, labels_test],
         axis=1).dropna(axis=0)


         for col in cluster_labels_train:
             cluster_labels_train[col] = cluster_labels_train[col].astype('category')

         for col in cluster_labels_test:
             cluster_labels_test[col] = cluster_labels_test[col].astype('category')

diastolic BP
Using 2352 ICU stays for creating the clusters
Using 1387 ICU stays for cluster assignment
4 clusters
Cluster 1: 633 observations
Cluster 2: 414 observations
Cluster 3: 658 observations
Cluster 4: 647 observations
```

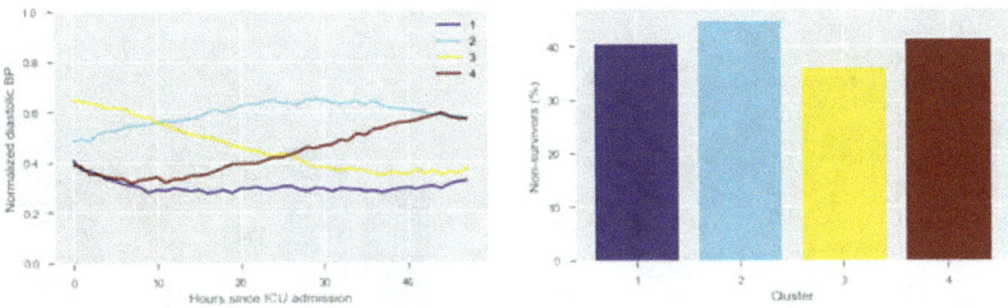

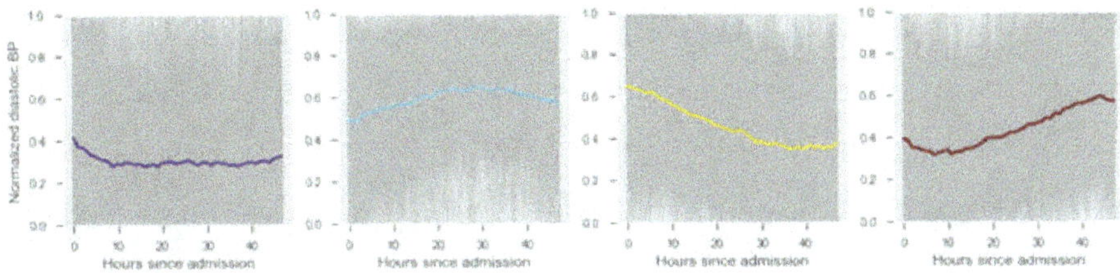


```
glucose
Using 2351 ICU stays for creating the clusters
Using 1387 ICU stays for cluster assignment
5 clusters
Cluster 1: 362 observations
Cluster 2: 716 observations
Cluster 3: 431 observations
Cluster 4: 398 observations
Cluster 5: 444 observations
```

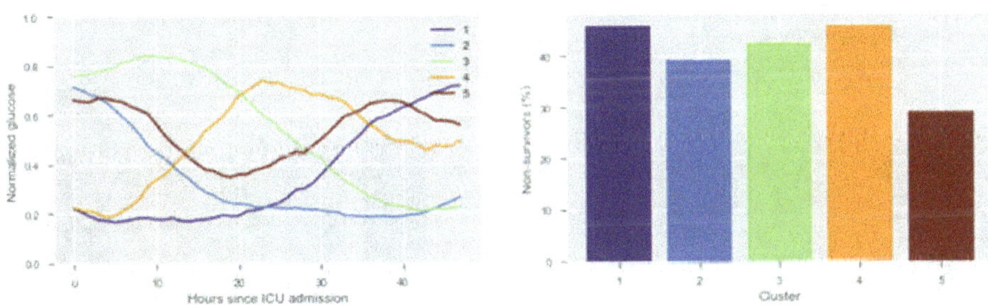

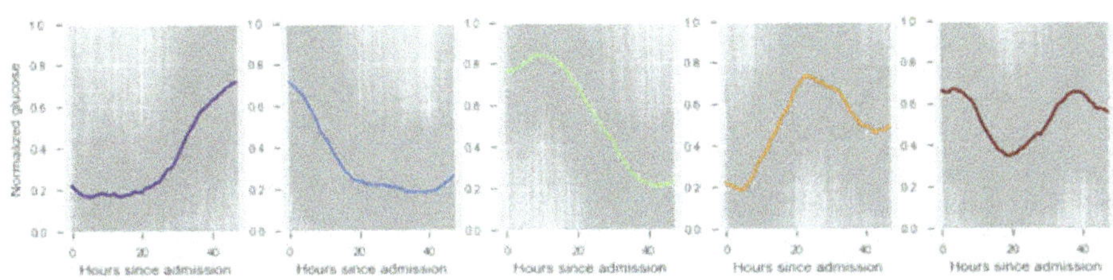


```
heart rate
Using 2350 ICU stays for creating the clusters
Using 1387 ICU stays for cluster assignment
5 clusters
Cluster 1: 455 observations
Cluster 2: 455 observations
```

```
Cluster 3: 452 observations
Cluster 4: 482 observations
Cluster 5: 506 observations
```

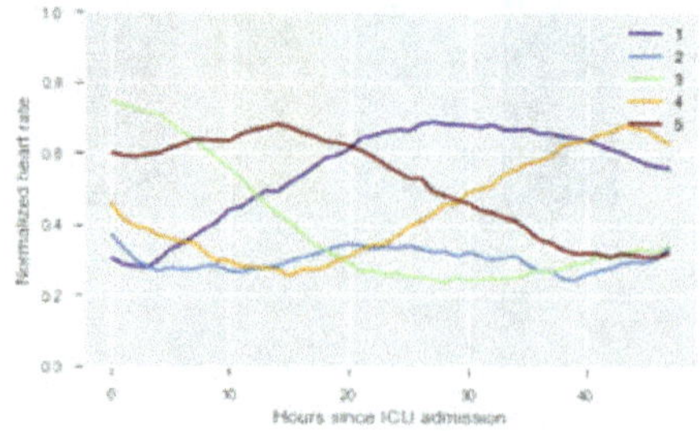

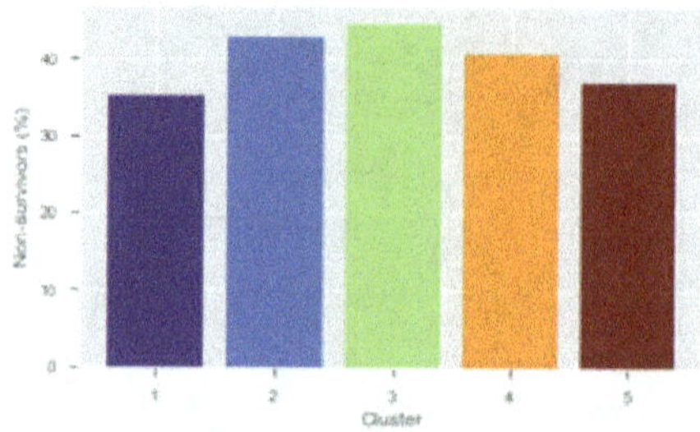

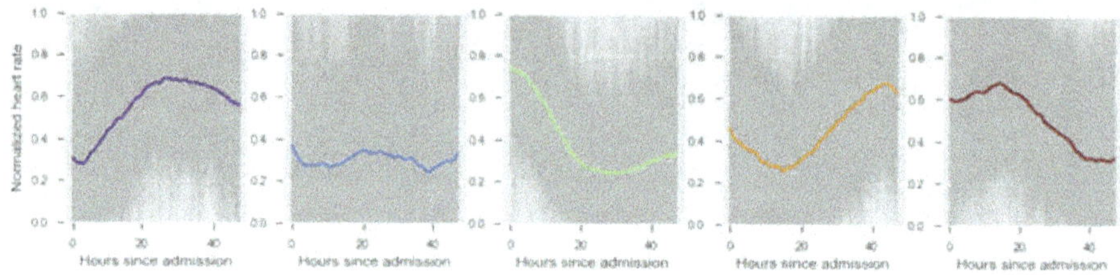


```
mean BP
Using 2352 ICU stays for creating the clusters
Using 1387 ICU stays for cluster assignment
5 clusters
Cluster 1: 505 observations
Cluster 2: 499 observations
Cluster 3: 526 observations
Cluster 4: 381 observations
Cluster 5: 441 observations
```

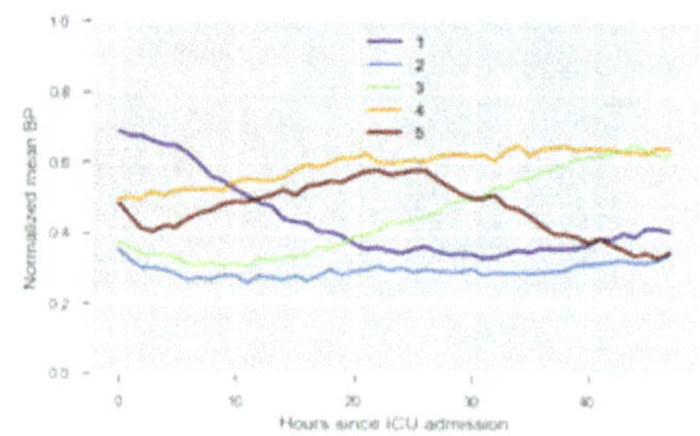

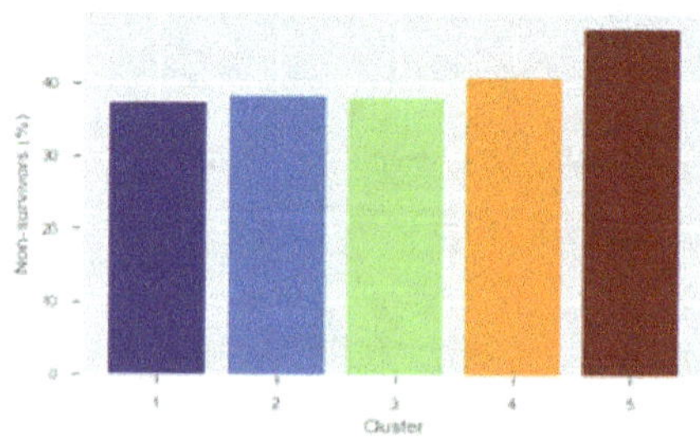

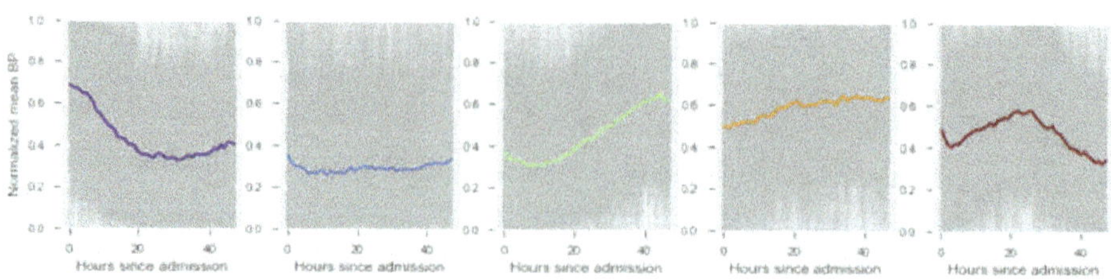


```
oxygen saturation
Using 2344 ICU stays for creating the clusters
Using 1378 ICU stays for cluster assignment
```

```
3 clusters
Cluster 1: 466 observations
Cluster 2: 1143 observations
Cluster 3: 735 observations
```

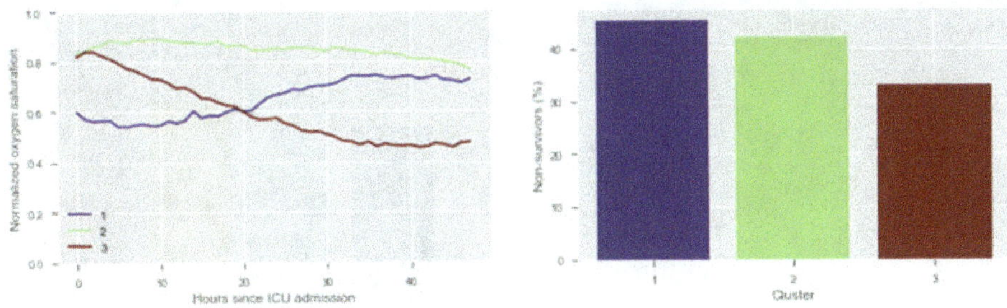

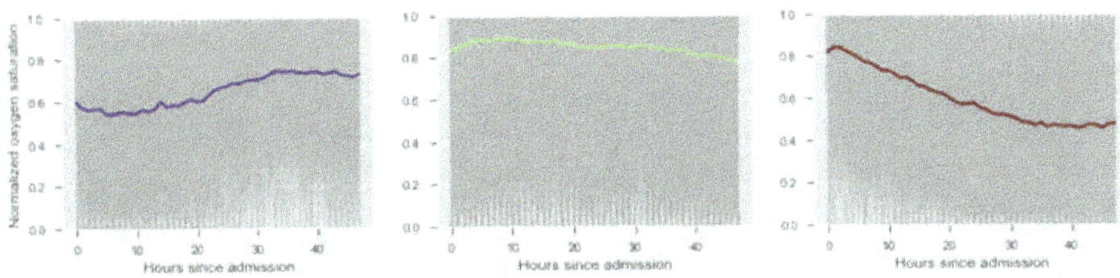


```
respiratory rate
Using 2352 ICU stays for creating the clusters
Using 1387 ICU stays for cluster assignment
5 clusters
Cluster 1: 385 observations
Cluster 2: 500 observations
Cluster 3: 516 observations
Cluster 4: 468 observations
Cluster 5: 483 observations
```

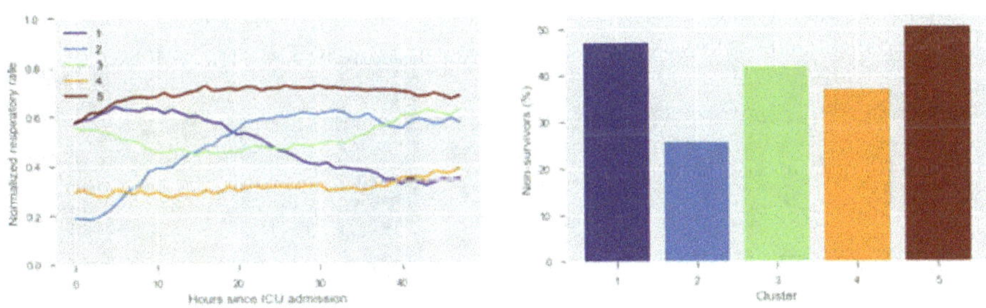

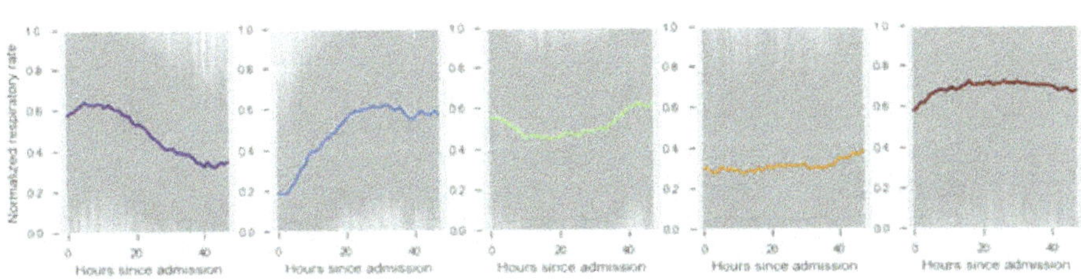


```
systolic BP
Using 2352 ICU stays for creating the clusters
```

```
Using 1387 ICU stays for cluster assignment
4 clusters
Cluster 1: 653 observations
Cluster 2: 586 observations
Cluster 3: 574 observations
Cluster 4: 539 observations
```

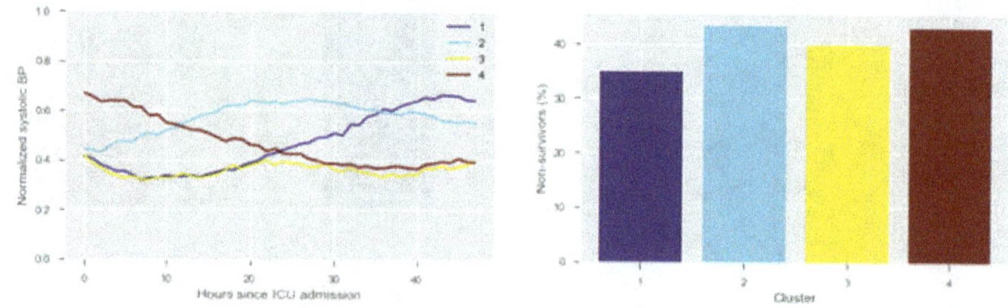

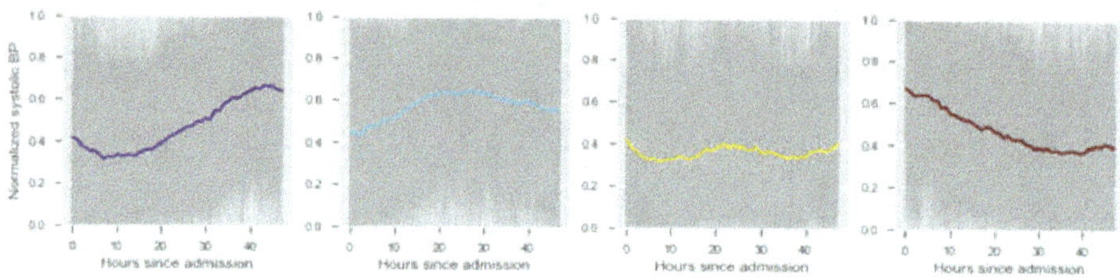


```
temperature
Using 2352 ICU stays for creating the clusters
Using 1387 ICU stays for cluster assignment
4 clusters
Cluster 1: 472 observations
Cluster 2: 695 observations
Cluster 3: 561 observations
Cluster 4: 624 observations
```

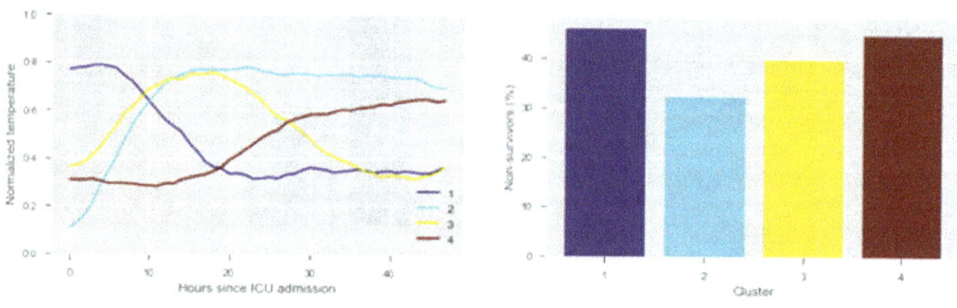

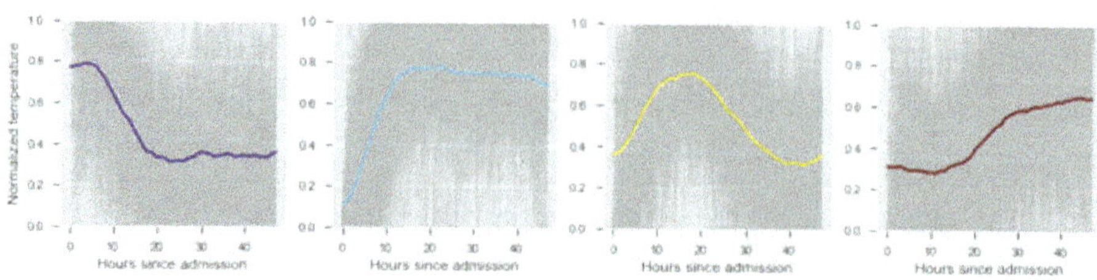

```
pH
Using 2326 ICU stays for creating the clusters
Using 1363 ICU stays for cluster assignment
4 clusters
Cluster 1: 472 observations
Cluster 2: 789 observations
Cluster 3: 643 observations
Cluster 4: 422 observations
```

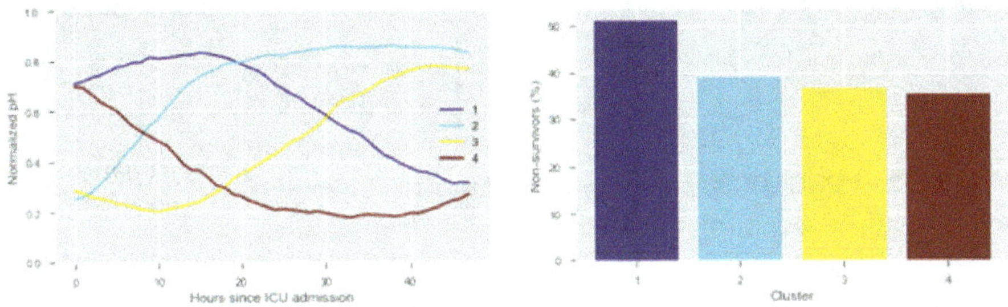

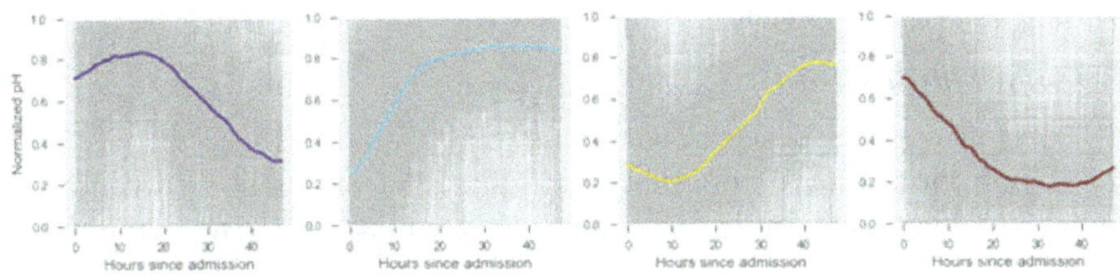

Clustering allowed us to stratify patients according to their physiological evolution during the first 48 h in the ICU. Since cluster centers reflect the cluster tendency, it is possible to investigate the relationship between distinct physiological patterns and mortality and ascertain to if the relationship is expected. For example, cluster 4 and cluster 5 in glucose are more or less symmetric: in cluster 4, patients start with low glucose, which increases over time until it decreases again; in cluster 5, patients start with high glucose, which decreases over time until it increases again. In the first case, mortality is approximately 45% and in the second case it is approximately 30%. Although this is obviously not enough to predict mortality, it highlights a possible relationship between the evolution of glucose and mortality. If a certain patient has a pattern of glucose similar to cluster 4, there may be more reason for concern than if they express the pattern in cluster 5.

By now, some particularities of the type of normalization performed can be noted:

- It hinders interpretability;
- It allows the algorithm to group together patients that did not present significant changes in their physiological state through time, regardless of the absolute value of the observations.

We have seen how clustering can be used to stratify patients, but not how it can be used to predict outcomes. Predictive models that use the information provided by clustering are investigated next. Models are created for the extracted features together with cluster information. This idea is represented in Fig. 10.1.

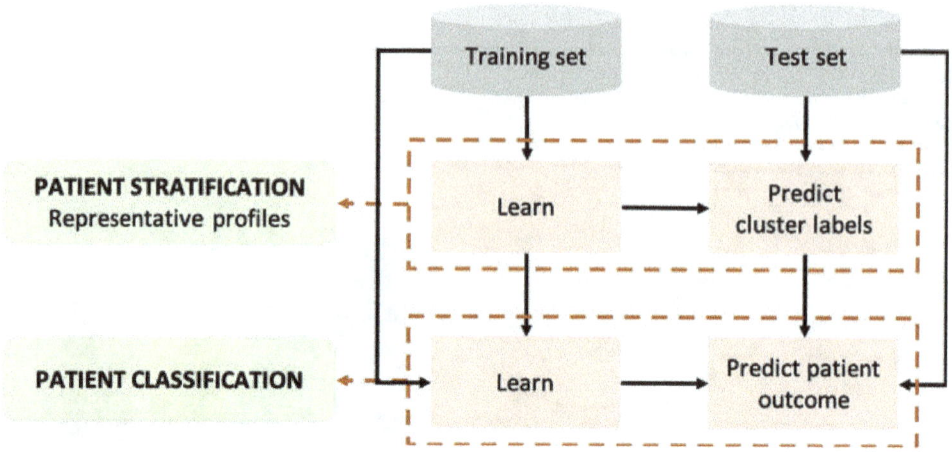

Fig. 10.1 Schematic representation of the machine learning steps

10.1.4 Normalization

Normalization, or scaling, is used to ensure that all features lie between a given minimum and maximum value, often between zero and one. The maximum and minimum values of each feature should be determined during the training phase and the same values should be applied during the test phase.

The next example is used to normalize the features extracted from the time series.

```
In [34]: X_train_min = X_train.min()
         X_train_max = X_train.max()
         X_train_norm = (X_train - X_train_min) / (X_train_max - X_train_min)
         X_test_norm = (X_test - X_train_min) / (X_train_max - X_train_min)
```

Normalization is useful when solving for example least squares or functions involving the calculation of distances. Contrary to what was done in clustering, the data is normalized for all patients together and not for each patient individually, i.e., the maximum and minimum values used for scaling are those found in the entire training set.

The next example uses the 'preprocessing' package from 'sklearn', which performs exactly the same:

```
In [35]: from sklearn import preprocessing

         min_max_scaler = preprocessing.MinMaxScaler()
         X_train_norm_skl = pd.DataFrame(min_max_scaler.fit_transform(X_train))

         # the same normalization operations will be applied to be consistent with the
         # transformation performed on the train data.
         X_test_norm_skl = pd.DataFrame(min_max_scaler.transform(X_test))
```

10.1.5 Concatenate Predicted Clustering Labels with Extracted Features

In the next example, the 'get_dummies' function from 'pandas' is used to get dummy variables for the cluster labels obtained through k-means. The idea is to use binary cluster labels, i.e., features indicating "yes/no belongs to cluster k", as input to the models. This will provide an extra level of information regarding the clinical temporal evolution of the patient in a multidimensional space.

You can add a 'drop_first' parameter to the 'get_dummies' function to indicate if you want to exclude one category, i.e., whether to get k–1 dummies out of k categorical levels by removing the first level. Because we will perform feature selection, this option does not need to be selected.

```
In [37]: # drop_first : bool, default False
         # use drop_first=True to exclude one of the categories

         X_train_clust = pd.get_dummies(cluster_labels_train, prefix_sep=' ')
         y_train_clust =
         pd.DataFrame(data_transf_inv.loc[cluster_labels_train.index]['mortality'])
         X_test_clust = pd.get_dummies(cluster_labels_test, prefix_sep=' ')
         y_test_clust = pd.DataFrame(data_transf_inv.loc[cluster_labels_test.index]['mortality'])

         X_train = pd.concat([X_train_norm, X_train_clust], axis=1).dropna(axis=0)
         y_train = y_train.loc[X_train.index]

         X_test = pd.concat([X_test_norm, X_test_clust], axis=1).dropna(axis=0)
         y_test = y_test.loc[X_test.index]
```

The next example prints the number of observations in the training and test sets, total number of features and a snapshot of the data.

```
In [38]: print('Number of observations in training set: ' + str(X_train.shape[0]))
         print('Number of observations in test set: ' + str(X_test.shape[0]))
         print('Number of features: ' + str(X_train.shape[1]))
         display.display(X_train.head())
```

```
Number of observations in training set: 2110
Number of observations in test set: 1232
Number of features: 85

          min diastolic BP  min glasgow coma scale  min glucose  \
icustay
200019.0          0.370370                0.250000     0.461864
200220.0          0.506173                0.250000     0.559322
200250.0          0.506173                0.333333     0.387712
200379.0          0.395062                0.000000     0.368644
200488.0          0.617284                0.500000     0.283898

          min heart rate  min mean BP  min oxygen saturation  \
icustay
200019.0        0.347107     0.630719                  0.950
200220.0        0.752066     0.705882                  0.970
200250.0        0.685950     0.552287                  0.960
200379.0        0.570248     0.513072                  0.930
200488.0        0.561983     0.637255                  0.895

          min respiratory rate  min systolic BP  min temperature    min pH  \
icustay
200019.0              0.366667         0.877551         0.760278  0.746479
200220.0              0.300000         0.761905         0.643836  0.563380
```

```
200250.0            0.016667         0.591837          0.739726  0.732394
200379.0            0.300000         0.605442          0.760278  0.788732
200488.0            0.100000         0.605442          0.842466  0.845070

          ...  CL systolic BP 2.0  CL systolic BP 3.0  \
icustay   ...
200019.0  ...                 0.0                 1.0
200220.0  ...                 1.0                 0.0
200250.0  ...                 1.0                 0.0
200379.0  ...                 0.0                 1.0
200488.0  ...                 0.0                 1.0

          CL temperature 0.0  CL temperature 1.0  CL temperature 2.0  \
icustay
200019.0                 1.0                 0.0                 0.0
200220.0                 1.0                 0.0                 0.0
200250.0                 0.0                 0.0                 0.0
200379.0                 0.0                 0.0                 1.0
200488.0                 0.0                 0.0                 1.0

          CL temperature 3.0  CL pH 0.0  CL pH 1.0  CL pH 2.0  CL pH 3.0
icustay
200019.0                 0.0        0.0        0.0        0.0        1.0
200220.0                 0.0        0.0        0.0        1.0        0.0
200250.0                 1.0        1.0        0.0        0.0        0.0
200379.0                 0.0        0.0        0.0        1.0        0.0
200488.0                 0.0        0.0        0.0        1.0        0.0

[5 rows x 85 columns]
```

The dataset is now composed of a mixture of summary statistics obtained through simple operations and clustering. Cluster labels are categorized as 'CL'. For example, 'CL 0.0' corresponds to cluster 1, 'CL 1.0' to cluster 2 and so on.

In the following "Part 3—Supervised Learning", classification models will be created in order to predict mortality.

Acknowledgements This work was supported by the Portuguese Foundation for Science & Technology, through IDMEC, under LAETA, project UID/EMS/50022/2019 and LISBOA-01-0145-FEDER-031474 supported by Programs Operational Regional de Lisboa by FEDER and FCT.

11

Machine Learning for Phenotyping: Learning Under Supervision

Cátia M. Salgado and Susana M. Vieira

Abstract Machine Learning for Phenotyping is composed of three chapters and aims to introduce clinicians to machine learning (ML). It provides a guideline through the basic concepts underlying machine learning and the tools needed to easily implement it using the Python programming language and Jupyter notebook documents. It is divided into three main parts: part 1—data preparation and analysis; part 2—unsupervised learning for clustering and part 3—supervised learning for classification.

Keywords Machine learning · Phenotyping · Data preparation · Data analysis · Unsupervised learning · Clustering · Supervised learning · Classification · Clinical informatics

11.1 Supervised Learning for Classification

The next section focuses on building mortality prediction models/classifiers using common algorithms and the 'sklearn' library, in particular k-nearest neighbors, logistic regression, decision trees and random forest. Before starting, it is important to define which performance measures should be used to evaluate the performance of different classifiers.

11.1.1 Definition of Performance Measures

Having a single-number evaluation metric is useful for comparing the performance of different models. Accuracy can be misleading when classes are imbalanced. Sensitivity (also called "recall" or "true positive rate") is a useful measure that indicates the percentage of non-survivors who are correctly identified as such. In the context

C. M. Salgado (✉) · S. M. Vieira
IDMEC, Instituto Superior Técnico, Universidade de Lisboa, Av. Rovisco Pais, Lisboa, Portugal
e-mail: catia.salgado@tecnico.ulisboa.pt

of our problem, having a high sensitivity is very important, since it tells us the algorithm is able to correctly identify the most critical cases. However, optimizing for sensitivity alone may lead to the presence of many false alarms (i.e. false positives). Therefore, it is important to also have in mind specificity, which tells us the percentage of survivors who are correctly identified. Sensitivity and specificity are given by:

- Sensitivity = $\frac{TP}{TP+FN}$
- Specificity = $\frac{TN}{TN+FP}$

One way of combining sensitivity and specificity in a single measure is using the area under the receiver-operator characteristics (ROC) curve (AUC), which is a graphical plot that illustrates the performance of a binary classifier as its discrimination threshold is varied.

The following function shows how to calculate the number of true positives, true negatives, false positives, false negatives, accuracy, sensitivity, specificity and AUC using the 'metrics' and 'confusion_matrix' packages from 'sklearn'; how to plot the ROC curve and how to choose a threshold in order to convert a continuous value output into a binary classification.

```
In [39]: from sklearn import metrics
         from sklearn.metrics import confusion_matrix

         def performance(y, y_pred, print_ = 1, *args):
             """ Calculate performance measures for a given ground truth classification y and
         predicted
             probabilities y_pred. If *args is provided a predifined threshold is used to
         calculate the performance.
             If not, the threshold giving the best mean sensitivity and specificity is selected.
         The AUC is calculated
             for a range of thresholds using the metrics package from sklearn. """

             # xx and yy values for ROC curve
             fpr, tpr, thresholds = metrics.roc_curve(y, y_pred, pos_label=1)
             # area under the ROC curve
             AUC = metrics.auc(fpr, tpr)

             if args:
                 threshold = args[0]
             else:
                 # we will choose the threshold that gives the best balance between sensitivity
and specificity
                 difference = abs((1-fpr) - tpr)
                 threshold = thresholds[difference.argmin()]

             # transform the predicted probability into a binary classification
             y_pred[y_pred >= threshold] = 1
             y_pred[y_pred < threshold] = 0

             tn, fp, fn, tp = confusion_matrix(y, y_pred).ravel()
             sensitivity = tp/(tp+fn)
             specificity = tn/(tn+fp)
             accuracy = (tp + tn) / (tp + tn + fp + fn)
```

```
    # print the performance and plot the ROC curve
    if print_ == 1:
        print('Threshold: ' + str(round(threshold,2)))
        print('TP: ' + str(tp))
        print('TN: ' + str(tn))
        print('FP: ' + str(fp))
        print('FN: ' + str(fn))
        print("Accuracy: " + str( round(accuracy, 2 )))
        print('Sensitivity: ' + str(round(sensitivity,2)))
        print('Specificity: ' + str(round(specificity,2)))
        print('AUC: ' + str(round(AUC,2)))

        plt.figure(figsize = (4,3))
        plt.scatter(x = fpr, y = tpr, label = None)
        plt.plot(fpr, tpr, label = 'Classifier', zorder = 1)
        plt.plot([0, 1], [0, 1], 'k--', label = 'Random classifier')
        plt.scatter(x = 1 - specificity, y = sensitivity, c = 'black', label =
'Operating point', zorder = 2)
        plt.legend()
        plt.xlabel('1 - specificity')
        plt.ylabel('sensitivity')
        plt.show()

    return threshold, AUC, sensitivity, specificity
```

11.1.2 Logistic Regression

When starting a machine learning project it is always a good approach to begin with a very simple model since it will give a sense of how challenging the question is. Logistic regression (LR) is considered a simple model because the underlying math is easy to understand, thus making its parameters and results interpretable. It also takes time computing compared to other ML models.

11.1.2.1 Feature Selection

In order to reduce multicollinearity, and because we are interested in increasing the interpretability and simplicity of the model, feature selection is highly recommended. Multicollinearity exists when two or more of the predictors in a regression model are moderately or highly correlated. The problem with multicollinearity is that it makes some variables statistically insignificant when they are not necessarily so, because the estimated coefficient of one variable depends on which collinear variables are included in the model. High multicollinearity increases the variance of the regression coefficients, making them unstable, but a little bit of multicollinearity is not necessarily a problem. As you will see, the algorithm used for feature selection does not directly addresses multicollinearity, but indirectly helps reduce it by reducing the size of the feature space.

Sequential forward selection/forward stepwise selection The sequential forward selection (SFS) algorithm is an iterative process where the subset of features that best predicts the output is obtained by sequentially selecting features until there is no improvement in prediction. The criterion used to select features and to determine when to stop is chosen based on the objectives of the problem. In this work, maximization of average sensitivity and specificity will be used as the criterion.

In the first iteration, models with one feature are created (univariable analysis). The model that yields the higher average sensitivity and specificity in the validation set is selected. In the second iteration, the remaining features are evaluated again one at a time, together with the feature selected in the previous iteration. This process continues until there is no significant improvement in performance.

In order to evaluate different feature sets, the training data is divided into two sets, one for training and another for validation. This can be easily achieved using the 'train_test_split' as before:

```
In [40]: val_size = 0.4
         X_train_SFS, X_val_SFS, y_train_SFS, y_val_SFS = train_test_split(X_train, y_train,
         test_size = val_size, random_state = 10)
```

Since there is no SFS implementation in python, the algorithm is implemented from scratch in the next example. The 'linear model' package from 'sklearn' is used to implement LR and a minimum improvement of 0.0005 is used in order to visualize the algorithm for a few iterations. The figure shows the performance associated with each feature at each iteration of the algorithm. Different iterations have different colors and at each iteration one feature is selected and marked with a red dot. Note that this operation will take some time to compute. You can decrease the 'min_improv' to visualize the algorithm for fewer iterations or increase it to allow more features to be added to the final set. You can also remove the lines of code for plotting the performance at each run, to reduce the time of computation.

```
In [42]: from sklearn.linear_model import LogisticRegression
         from matplotlib import cm

         min_improv = 0.0005

         to_test_features = X_train_SFS.columns
         selected_features_sfs = []
         test_set = []
         results_selected = []
         previous_perf = 0
         gain = 1
         it = 0

         # create figure
         plt.figure(num=None, figsize=(15, 6))
         plt.xticks(rotation='vertical', horizontalalignment='right')
         plt.ylabel('Average sensitivity specificity')
         colors = cm.tab20(np.linspace(0, 1, 180))
         # just make sure you select an interval that gives you enough colors
         colors = colors[::10]

         # perform SFS while there is a gain in performance
         while gain >= min_improv:
             frames = []
             color = colors[it]
             it += 1
```

```
        # add one feature at a time to the previously selected feature set.
        for col in to_test_features:
            test_set = selected_features_sfs.copy()
            test_set.append(col)

            # train model
            model = LogisticRegression(random_state = 1)
            model.fit(X_train_SFS[test_set], y_train_SFS.values.ravel())

            # test performance
            y_pred_prob = model.predict_proba(X_val_SFS[test_set])
            _, AUC, sens, spec = performance(y_val_SFS, np.delete(y_pred_prob, 0, 1), print_
= 0)

            # save the results
            frames.append([test_set, (sens+spec)/2])

            # plot the performance
            plt.scatter(x = col, y = (sens+spec)/2, c = color)
            display.display(plt.gcf())
            display.clear_output(wait=True)
            time.sleep(0.001)

        # select best feature combination
        results = pd.DataFrame(frames, columns=('Feature', 'Performance'))
        id_max = results.loc[results['Performance'].idxmax()]
        gain = id_max['Performance'] - previous_perf

        # plot selected feature combination in red
        plt.scatter(x = id_max['Feature'][-1], y = id_max['Performance'], c = 'red', s =
150)

        # test if selected feature combination improves the performance
'min_improv'
        if gain > min_improv:
            previous_perf = id_max['Performance']
            to_test_features = to_test_features.drop(id_max['Feature'][-1])
            selected_features_sfs.append(id_max['Feature'][-1])
            results_selected.append(id_max)
        # if not, do not had the last feature to the feature set. Exit the loop

    results_selected = pd.DataFrame(results_selected)
```

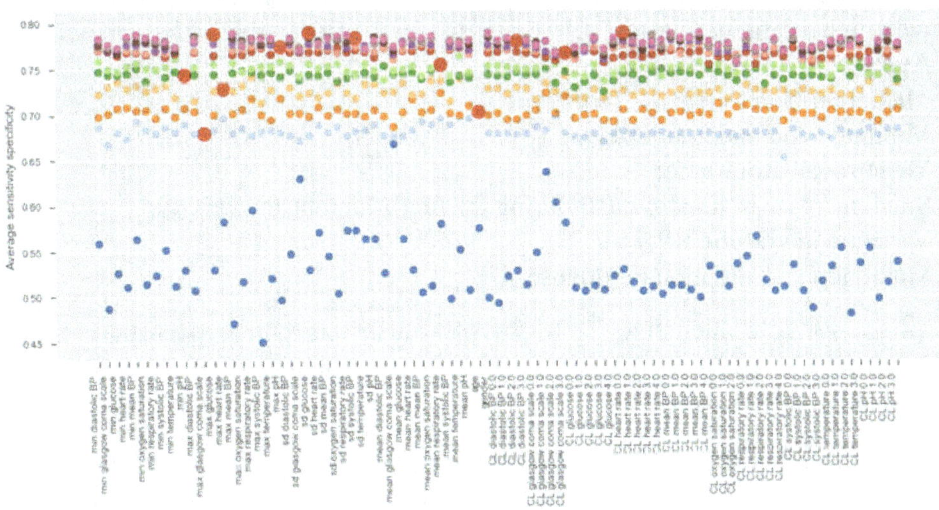

Iteration 1 (blue dots associated with lower performance) corresponds to a univariable analysis. At this stage, maximum GCS is selected since it yields the higher average sensitivity and specificity. Iteration 2 corresponds to a multivariable analysis (GCS plus every other independent variable). There is a big jump from iteration 1 to iteration 2, as expected, and small improvements thereafter until the performance reaches a plateau. We can plot the performance obtained at each iteration:

```
In [43]: plt.figure(num=None, figsize=(10, 4))
         plt.scatter(x = range(1,results_selected.shape[0]+1,1), y =
         results_selected['Performance'], c = 'red', s = 150)
         plt.xticks(range(1,results_selected.shape[0]+1,1),results_selected['Feature'].iloc[-1],
         rotation = 'vertical')
         plt.ylabel('AUC')
         plt.show()
```

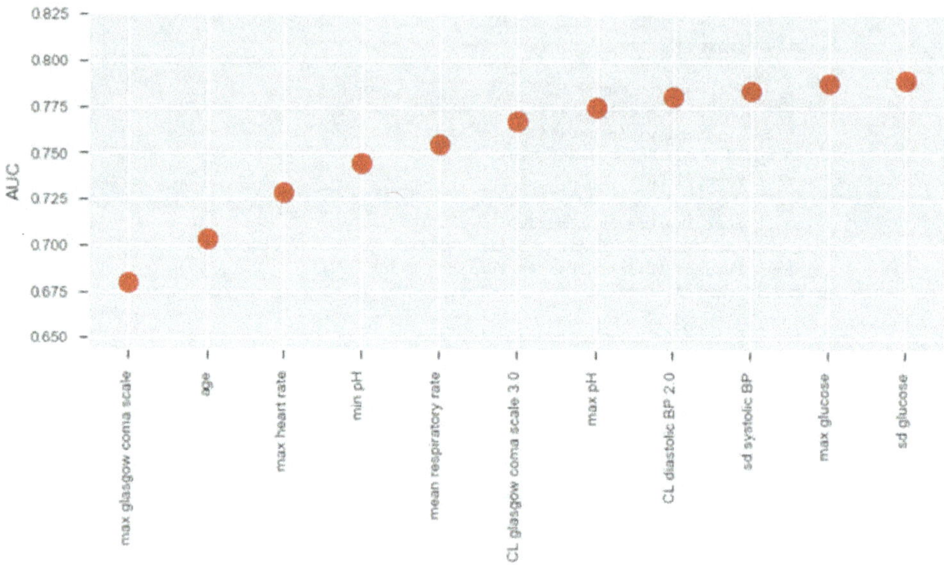

According to SFS, important features that help predict the outcome are:

- Maximum **GCS**, decrease in **GCS** during the first hours in the ICU associated with high mortality (cluster 3);
- **Age**;
- Maximum **heart rate**;
- Minimum and maximum **pH**;
- Mean **respiratory rate**;
- Small increase in **diastolic BP** during the first 24 h (cluster 2);
- Variation in **systolic BP**;
- Maximum and variation in **glucose**.

In the exercises you will be advised to investigate how these conclusions change when a different data partitioning is used for training and testing. You can do this by changing the random seed.

Remember that for large number of features (85 in our case) we cannot compute the best subset sequence. This would mean testing all combinations of 85 features, 1–85 at a time. It is hard enough to calculate the number of combinations, let alone train models for every one of them. This is why greedy algorithms that lead to sub-optimal solutions are commonly used. Even k-means, which is very fast (one of the fastest clustering algorithms available), falls in local minima.

Recursive Feature Elimination (RFE) Recursive feature elimination is similar to forward stepwise selection, only in this case features are recursively eliminated (as opposed to being recursively added) from the feature set. It can be implemented using the 'RFE' function from 'sklearn'. At the 'sklearn' documentation website you will find:

"Given an external estimator that assigns weights to features (e.g., the coefficients of a linear model), the goal of recursive feature elimination (RFE) is to select features by recursively considering smaller and smaller sets of features. First, the estimator is trained on the initial set of features and the importance of each feature is obtained either through a 'coef_' attribute or through a 'feature_importances_' attribute. Then, the least important features are pruned from current set of features. That procedure is recursively repeated on the pruned set until the desired number of features to select is eventually reached."

A disadvantage of using 'sklearn' implementation of RFE is that you are limited to using 'coef_' or 'feature_importances_' attributes to recursively exclude features. Since LR retrieves a 'coef_' attribute, this means RFE will recursively eliminate features that have low coefficients and not the features that yield the lower average sensitivity specificity as we would like to if we were to follow the example previously given with SFS.

Similarly to SFS, a stopping criterion must also be defined. In this case, the stopping criterion is the number of features. If the number of features is not given ('n_features_to_select' = None), half of the features are automatically selected. For illustrative purposes, the next example shows how to use RFE to select 13 features:

```
In [44]: from sklearn.feature_selection import RFE

         n_features_to_select = 13

         logreg = LogisticRegression(random_state = 1)
         rfe = RFE(logreg, n_features_to_select)
         rfe = rfe.fit(X_train, y_train.values.ravel())
```

The attribute 'support_' gives a mask of selected features:

```
In [45]: selected_features_rfe = X_train.columns[rfe.support_]

         print('Number of features selected: ' + str(len(X_selected_features_rfe)))
         print()
         print('Selected features:')
         display.display(selected_features_rfe)
```

```
Number of features selected: 13

Selected features:

Index(['min diastolic BP', 'min heart rate', 'min mean BP', 'max heart rate',
       'sd glasgow coma scale', 'sd oxygen saturation', 'sd temperature',
```

```
 'sd pH', 'mean glasgow coma scale', 'mean glucose',
 'mean respiratory rate', 'mean temperature', 'age'],
dtype='object')
```

The attribute 'ranking_' gives the feature ranking. Features are ranked according to when they were eliminated and selected features are assigned rank 1:

```
In [46]: rfe.ranking_
```

```
Out[46]: array([ 1, 52,  6,  1,  1, 64, 20, 31, 43, 11, 16,  3, 72,  1, 19,  5,  9,
               26, 46, 57, 45,  1, 24,  8, 13,  1, 14,  7,  1,  1, 10,  1,  1, 15,
               32, 30,  1, 53,  1, 38,  1, 51, 37, 35, 68, 36, 40, 39,  4,  2, 17,
               73, 69, 25, 67, 50, 48, 41, 49, 70, 60, 61, 63, 62, 18, 27, 28, 29,
               65, 66, 42, 47, 58, 71, 33, 44, 34, 22, 59, 21, 23, 12, 56, 55, 54])
```

For example, the last feature to be excluded by RFE is:

```
In [47]: X_train.columns[rfe.ranking_.argmax()]
```

```
Out[47]: 'CL glucose 1.0'
```

However, this does not mean that this particular cluster tendency of glucose is not important; such a conclusion cannot be drawn due to the presence of other features that are highly correlated with this one.

SFS and RFE selected the following features in common:

```
In [48]: list(set(selected_features_rfe) & set(selected_features_sfs))
```

```
Out[48]: ['age', 'mean respiratory rate', 'max heart rate']
```

11.1.2.2 Model Testing

Feature selection has been performed using training and validation sets. In the next steps, the performance is evaluated using an independent test set not used to select features. First, a LR model is fitted to the training data on the feature set selected by SFS:

```
In [49]: model = LogisticRegression(random_state = 1)
         model.fit(X_train[selected_features_sfs], y_train.values.ravel())
```

```
Out[49]: LogisticRegression(C=1.0, class_weight=None, dual=False, fit_intercept=True,
                  intercept_scaling=1, max_iter=100, multi_class='ovr', n_jobs=1,
                  penalty='l2', random_state=1, solver='liblinear', tol=0.0001,
                  verbose=0, warm_start=False)
```

Next, a general function called 'model_evaluation' is created in order to:

1. yield probability estimates for unseen data. This is achieved using the 'predict_proba' function;
2. evaluate model performance using both training and test sets.

```
In [50]: def model_evaluation(model, X_train, y_train, X_test, y_test, print_):

             # tune - parameter estimation
             print('TRAINING SET')
             y_pred_prob_train = model.predict_proba(X_train)
             threshold, AUC_train, sens_train, spec_train = performance(y_train,
         np.delete(y_pred_prob_train, 0, 1), print_)

             # test
             print('TEST SET')
             y_pred_prob_test = model.predict_proba(X_test)
             _, AUC_test, sens_test, spec_test = performance(y_test, np.delete(y_pred_prob_test,
         0, 1), print_, threshold)

             # save the results
             results_train = pd.DataFrame(data = [[threshold, AUC_train, sens_train, spec_train,
         X_train.shape[1]]],
                                        columns = ['Threshold','AUC', 'Sensitivity', 'Specificity',
         '# features'])

             results_test = pd.DataFrame(data = [[threshold, AUC_test, sens_test, spec_test,
         X_train.shape[1]]],
                                        columns = ['Threshold','AUC', 'Sensitivity', 'Specificity',
         '# features'])

             return results_train, results_test, y_pred_prob_train, y_pred_prob_test
```

We can call the function to evaluate the previous model on test data:

```
In [51]: results_train, results_test, y_pred_prob_train, y_pred_prob_test =
         model_evaluation(model, X_train[selected_features_sfs], y_train,
         X_test[selected_features_sfs], y_test, print_ = 1)
```

```
TRAINING SET
Threshold: 0.39
TP: 631
TN: 970
FP: 308
FN: 201
Accuracy: 0.76
Sensitivity: 0.76
Specificity: 0.76
AUC: 0.82
```

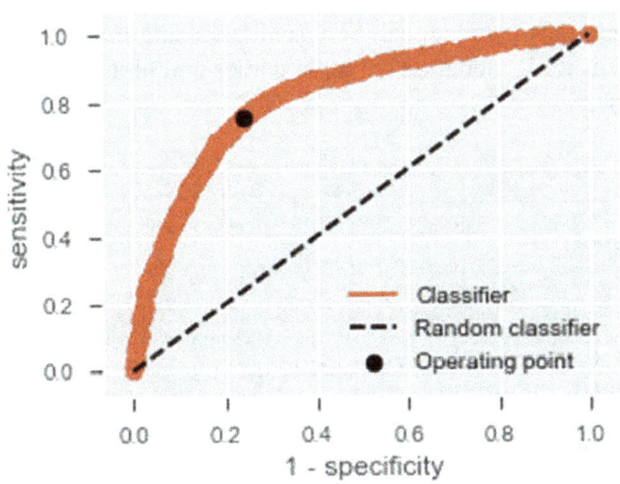

```
TEST SET
Threshold: 0.39
TP: 158
TN: 727
FP: 283
FN: 64
Accuracy: 0.72
Sensitivity: 0.71
Specificity: 0.72
AUC: 0.79
```

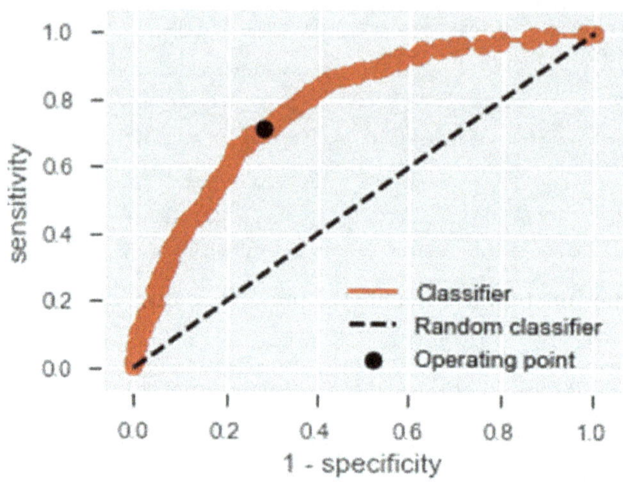

Results are assigned to a DataFrame for future reference, with the label 'LR SFS':

```
In [52]: all_results_train = pd.DataFrame()
         all_results_test = pd.DataFrame()
         all_results_train =
         all_results_train.append(results_train.rename(index={results_train.index[-1]: 'LR
         SFS'}))
         all_results_test =
         all_results_test.append(results_test.rename(index={results_test.index[-1]: 'LR SFS'}))
```

The coefficients of the model can be visualized using the 'coef_' attribute. The next function takes a LR model and column names and plots the model coefficients in ascending order:

```
In [53]: def print_coef(model, columns):
             """ Plot logistic regression model coefficients """
             coef = pd.DataFrame(np.transpose(model.coef_), index = columns, columns =
         ['Coefficients'])
             coef = coef.sort_values(by=['Coefficients'])
             plt.figure(figsize = (15,6))
             plt.scatter(x = range(len(coef)), y = coef['Coefficients'])
             plt.xticks(range(len(coef)),coef.index, rotation = 'vertical')
             plt.ylabel('LR coefficients')
             plt.show()
```

```
In [54]: print_coef(model, X_train[selected_features_sfs].columns)
```

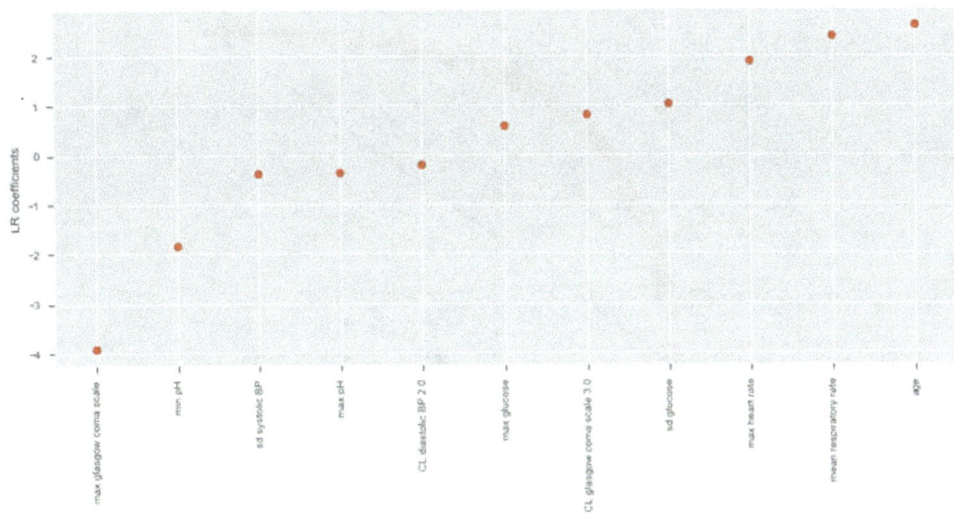

The results seem to cohere with expected clinical practice. There are enough variables in the model which correlate with mortality as we would expect them to. This increases our faith in the remainder of those variables whose association with mortality in clinical practice is not inherently obvious. The results evoke interesting relationships between other variables which are less well known to affect mortality, such as glucose.

The same process can be repeated for RFE:

```
In [55]: model = LogisticRegression(random_state = 1)
         model.fit(X_train[selected_features_rfe], y_train.values.ravel())
         results_train, results_test, y_pred_prob_train, y_pred_prob_test =
         model_evaluation(model, X_train[selected_features_rfe], y_train,
         X_test[selected_features_rfe], y_test, print_ = 1)
         print_coef(model, X_train[selected_features_rfe].columns)

         all_results_train =
         all_results_train.append(results_train.rename(index={results_train.index[-1]: 'LR
         RFE'}))
         all_results_test =
         all_results_test.append(results_test.rename(index={results_test.index[-1]: 'LR RFE'}))
```

```
TRAINING SET
Threshold: 0.4
TP: 638
TN: 981
FP: 297
FN: 194
Accuracy: 0.77
Sensitivity: 0.77
Specificity: 0.77
AUC: 0.85
```

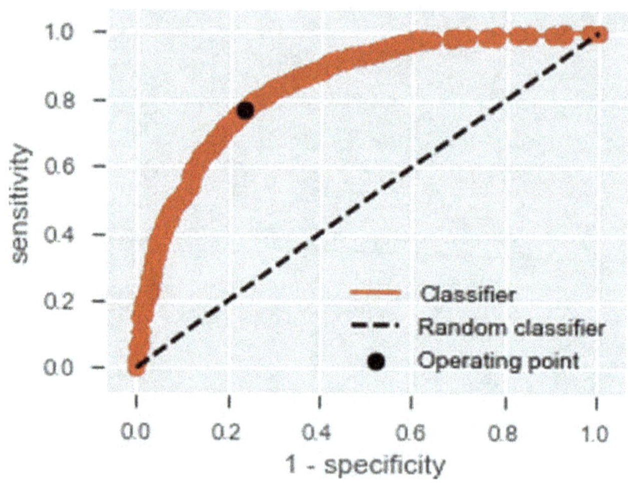


```
TEST SET
Threshold: 0.4
TP: 162
TN: 751
FP: 259
FN: 60
Accuracy: 0.74
Sensitivity: 0.73
Specificity: 0.74
AUC: 0.82
```

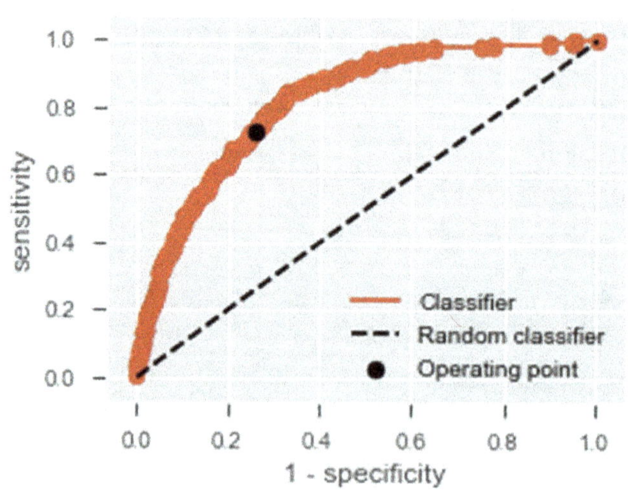

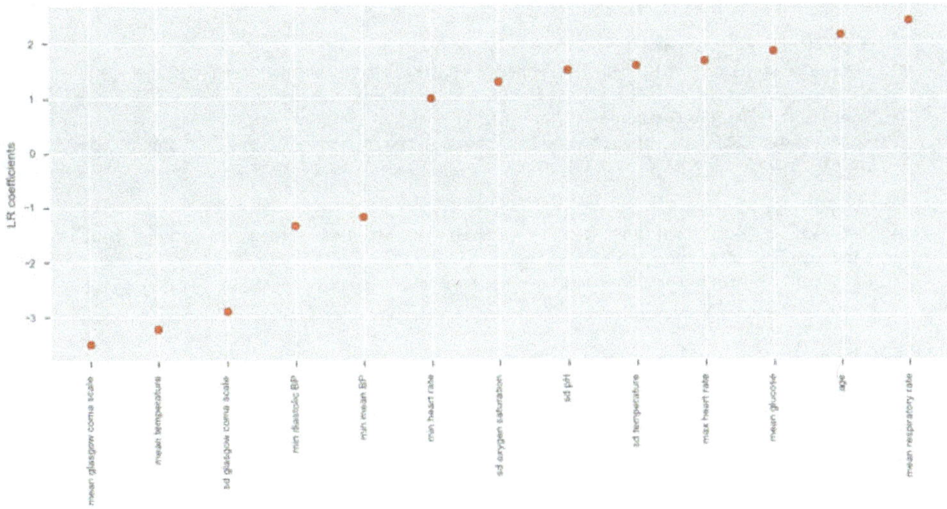

11.1.3 K-Nearest Neighbors

Another simple algorithm investigated in this work is k-nearest neighbors (kNN). It is known as a "lazy" algorithm, since it does not do anything during the learning phase: the model is essentially the entire training dataset. When a prediction is required for an unseen observation, kNN will search through the entire training set for the k most similar observations. The prediction is given by the majority voting of those k nearest neighbors. The similarity measure is dependent on the type of data. For real-valued data, the Euclidean distance can be used. For other types of data, such as categorical or binary data, the Hamming distance is recommended. In this work we focus only on the Euclidean distance.

A very common alternative to the straightforward kNN is weighted kNN, where each point has a weight proportional to its distance. For example, with inverse distance weighting, each point has a weight equal to the inverse of its distance to the point to be classified. This means that neighboring points have a higher vote than farther points. As an example, we will use the 'KNeighborsClassifier' function from 'sklearn' with 3 neighbors, with the parameter 'weights' set to 'distance', in order to have weighted votes and the features selected through SFS.

Warning: In 'sklearn', if there is a tie in majority voting, for instance if you provide $k = 2$ and the two neighbors have identical distances but different class labels, the results will depend on the ordering of the training data. Therefore, it is recommended to use an odd number of k.

```
In [56]: from sklearn.neighbors import KNeighborsClassifier

         # instantiate learning model
         knn = KNeighborsClassifier(n_neighbors = 3, weights = 'distance')

         # fitting the model
         knn.fit(X_train[selected_features_sfs], y_train.values.ravel())
```

```
# predict the response
y_pred = knn.predict(X_test[selected_features_sfs])

# evaluate the performance
threshold, AUC_test, sens_test, spec_test = performance(y_test, pd.DataFrame(y_pred),
print_ = 1)

# save the results
all_results_test.loc['KNN SFS'] = [threshold, AUC_test, sens_test, spec_test,
len(selected_features_sfs)]
all_results_train.loc['KNN SFS'] = np.nan
```

```
Threshold: 1
TP: 125
TN: 816
FP: 194
FN: 97
Accuracy: 0.76
Sensitivity: 0.56
Specificity: 0.81
AUC: 0.69
```

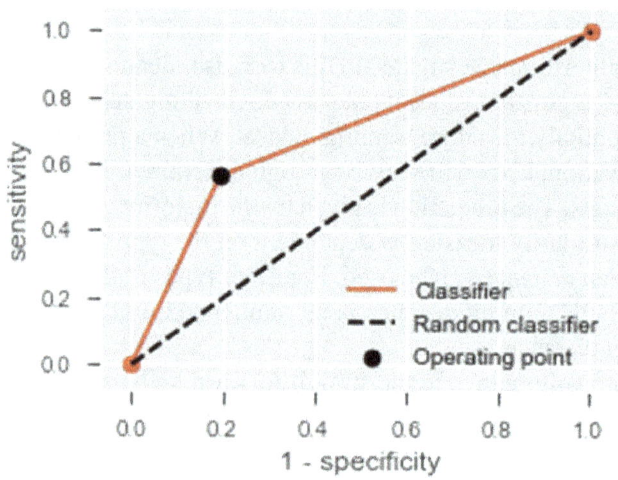

Running the same algorithm with the features selected through RFE yields very similar results. You can check for yourself by substituting the input vector in the previous script.

11.1.4 Decision Tree

Most ICU severity scores are constructed using logistic regression, which imposes stringent constraints on the relationship between explanatory variables and the outcome. In particular, logistic regression relies on the assumption of a linear and additive relationship between the outcome and its predictors. Given the complexity of the processes underlying death in ICU patients, this assumption might be unrealistic.

We hope to improve the prediction obtained by LR by using a nonparametric algorithm such as a decision tree (DT). A DT is a model that uses a tree-like graph of rules that provides probabilities of outcome. It can be used for classification and regression, it automatically performs feature selection, it is easy to understand, interpret (as long as the tree has a small depth and low number of features) and requires little data preparation. Since this type of algorithm does not make strong assumptions about the form of the mapping function, it is a good candidate when you have a lot of data and no prior knowledge, and when you do not want to worry too much about choosing the right features.

However, DT learners are associated with several disadvantages. They are prone to overfitting, as they tend to create over-complex trees that do not generalize well and they can be unstable because small variations in the data might result in a completely different tree being generated. Methods like bagging and boosting (i.e., random forests), are typically used to solve these issues.

11.1.4.1 CART Algorithm

This work will focus on the CART algorithm, which is one of the most popular algorithms for learning a DT. The selection of variables and the specific split is chosen using a greedy algorithm to minimize a cost function. Tree construction ends using a predefined stopping criterion, such as a minimum number of training instances assigned to each leaf node of the tree.

Greedy Splitting The greedy search consists of recursive binary splitting, a process of dividing up the input space. All input variables and all possible split points are evaluated and chosen in a greedy manner (the very best split point is chosen each time). All values are lined up and different split points are tried and tested using a cost function. The split with the lowest cost is selected.

For classification, the **Gini index** (G) function (also known as Gini impurity) is used. It provides an indication of how "pure" the leaf nodes are, or in other words, an idea of how good a split is by how mixed the classes are in the two groups created by the split:

- **perfect class purity**: a node that has all classes of the same ($G = 0$)
- **worst class purity**: a node that has a 50–50 split of classes ($G = 0.5$)

The G for each node is weighted by the total number of instances in the parent node. For a chosen split point in a binary classification problem, G is calculated as: $G = ((1 - g1_1^2 + g1_2^2) \times \frac{ng1}{n}) + ((1 - g2_1^2 + g2_2^2) \times \frac{ng2}{n})$, where:

- $g1_1$: proportion of instances in group 1 for class 1;
- $g1_2$: proportion of instances in group 1 for class 2;
- $g2_1$: proportion of instances in group 2 for class 1;
- $g2_2$: proportion of instances in group 2 for class 2;

- $ng1$: total number of instances in group 1;
- $ng2$: total number of instances in group 2;
- n: total number of instances we are trying to group from the parent node.

Stopping Criterion The most common stopping procedure is to use a minimum count of the number of training observations assigned to each leaf node. If the count is less than some minimum then the split is not accepted and the node is taken as a final leaf node. The minimum count of training observations is tuned to the dataset. It defines how specific to the training data the tree will be. Too specific (e.g. a count of 1) and the tree will overfit the training data and likely have poor performance on the test set.

The CART algorithm can be implemented in 'sklearn' using the 'DecisionTreeClassifier' function from sklearn.ensemble'. Next follows a list of important parameters to have in consideration when training the model:

- **criterion**: function to measure the quality of a split. Default = 'gini'.
- **splitter**: strategy used to choose the split at each node. Supported strategies are 'best' to choose the best split and 'random' to choose the best random split. Default = 'best'.
- **max_features**: maximum number of features in each tree. Default is sqrt(n_features).
- **max_depth**: maximum depth of the tree. If None, nodes are expanded until all leaves are pure or until all leaves contain less than 'min_samples_split' samples.
- **min_samples_split**: minimum number of samples required to split an internal node. Default = 2.
- **min_samples_leaf**: minimum number of samples required to be at a leaf node. Default = 1.
- **max_leaf_nodes**: grow a tree with 'max_leaf_nodes' in best-first fashion. Best nodes are defined as relative reduction in impurity. If None then unlimited number of leaf nodes. Default = None.
- **random_state**: if int, seed used by the random number generator. Default = None.

In the next example, a small DT (maximum depth of 5) is created. Since the algorithm has embedded feature selection, we can use all the extracted features as input without having to worry about dimensionality issues.

```
In [57]: # from sklearn import tree
         from sklearn.tree import DecisionTreeClassifier

         clf_gini = DecisionTreeClassifier(criterion = 'gini', max_depth = 5, min_samples_leaf =
         20,
                                           min_samples_split = 20, random_state = 2, splitter =
         'best')

         clf_gini.fit(X_train, y_train)
         results_train, results_test, y_pred_prob_train, y_pred_prob_test =
         model_evaluation(clf_gini, X_train, y_train, X_test, y_test, print_ = 1)
```

```
TRAINING SET
Threshold: 0.44
TP: 683
TN: 981
```

```
FP: 297
FN: 149
Accuracy: 0.79
Sensitivity: 0.82
Specificity: 0.77
AUC: 0.87
```

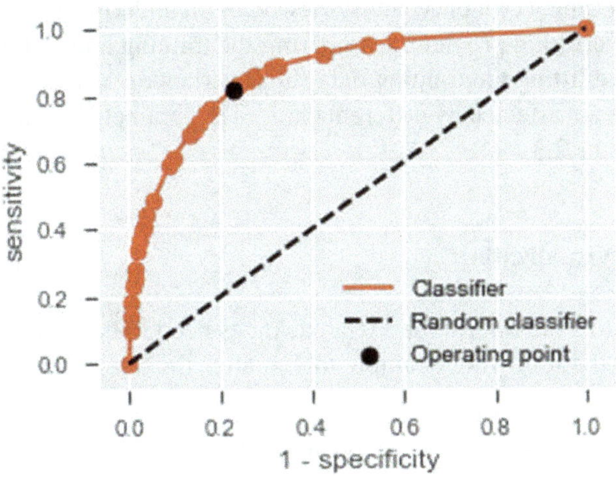


```
TEST SET
Threshold: 0.44
TP: 159
TN: 705
FP: 305
FN: 63
Accuracy: 0.7
Sensitivity: 0.72
Specificity: 0.7
AUC: 0.77
```

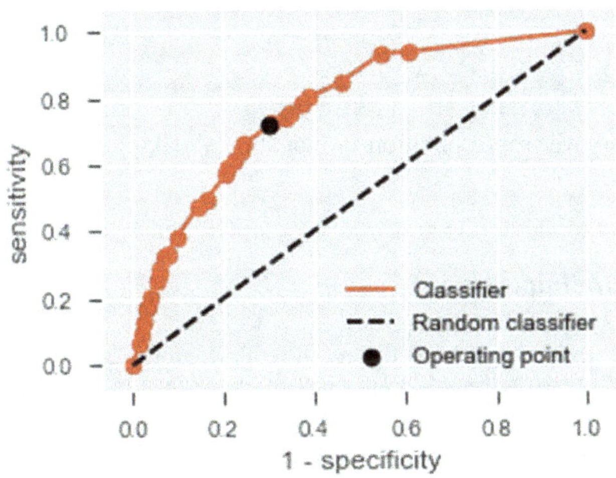

As already discussed in the previous Chapter, there are two major sources of error in machine learning—bias and variance:

- **Bias**: how the algorithm performs on the training set.
- **Variance**: how much worse the algorithm does on the test set than the training set.

Understanding them will help you decide which tactics to improve performance are a good use of time. High bias can be viewed as an underfitting problem and high variance as an overfitting problem. Comparing the training and test results, it seems that the DT is overfitting the training data (high variance). You can investigate how bias and variance are affected by different choices of parameters. This topic is further explored in Sect. 11.2.3.

11.1.4.2 Tree Visualization

In order to visualize the tree, some extra packages need to be installed ('pydot' and 'graphviz'). Use the following example to visualize the tree created in the previous step:

```
In [58]: from sklearn.externals.six import StringIO
         from IPython.display import Image
         from sklearn.tree import export_graphviz
         import pydotplus

         dot_data = StringIO()
         export_graphviz(clf_gini, out_file=dot_data,
                         filled=True, rounded=True,
                         special_characters=True,
                         class_names=["survival", "non-survival"],
                         feature_names=X_train.columns)
         graph = pydotplus.graph_from_dot_data(dot_data.getvalue())
         Image(graph.create_png())
```

Out[58]:

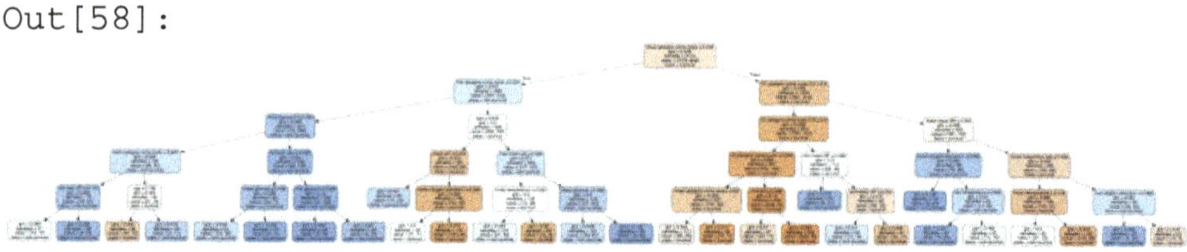

With the binary tree representation shown above, making predictions is relatively straightforward.

11.1.4.3 Feature Importance

As you can see in the previous figure, not all features are selected. The 'feature_importances_' attribute gives the relative importance of each feature in the model. The importance of a feature is computed as the (normalized) total reduction of the criterion yielded by that feature. It is also known as the Gini importance. Features with relative importance greater than 0 correspond to features that were selected by the model. The next example shows how to plot the features in descending order of relative importance.

```
In [59]: def plot_feat_importance(columns, feature_importances_, *topx):
             list_feat = list(zip(columns, feature_importances_))
             pd_list_feat = pd.DataFrame(list_feat)
             pd_list_feat.columns = ('Feature','Importance')
             pd_list_feat = pd_list_feat.sort_values(by='Importance')
             pd_list_feat = pd_list_feat[pd_list_feat['Importance']>0]

             if topx:
                 pd_list_top = pd_list_feat.iloc[topx[0]:]
             else:
                 pd_list_top = pd_list_feat
             plt.figure(figsize=(10,10))
             plt.scatter(y = range(len(pd_list_top)), x = pd_list_top['Importance'])
             plt.yticks(range(len(pd_list_top)),pd_list_top['Feature'])
             plt.title("Relative feature importance of features in decision tree classifier", ha
         = 'right')
             plt.xlabel("Relative feature importance")
             plt.show()
             return pd_list_top

         pd_list_top = plot_feat_importance(X_train.columns, clf_gini.feature_importances_)
```

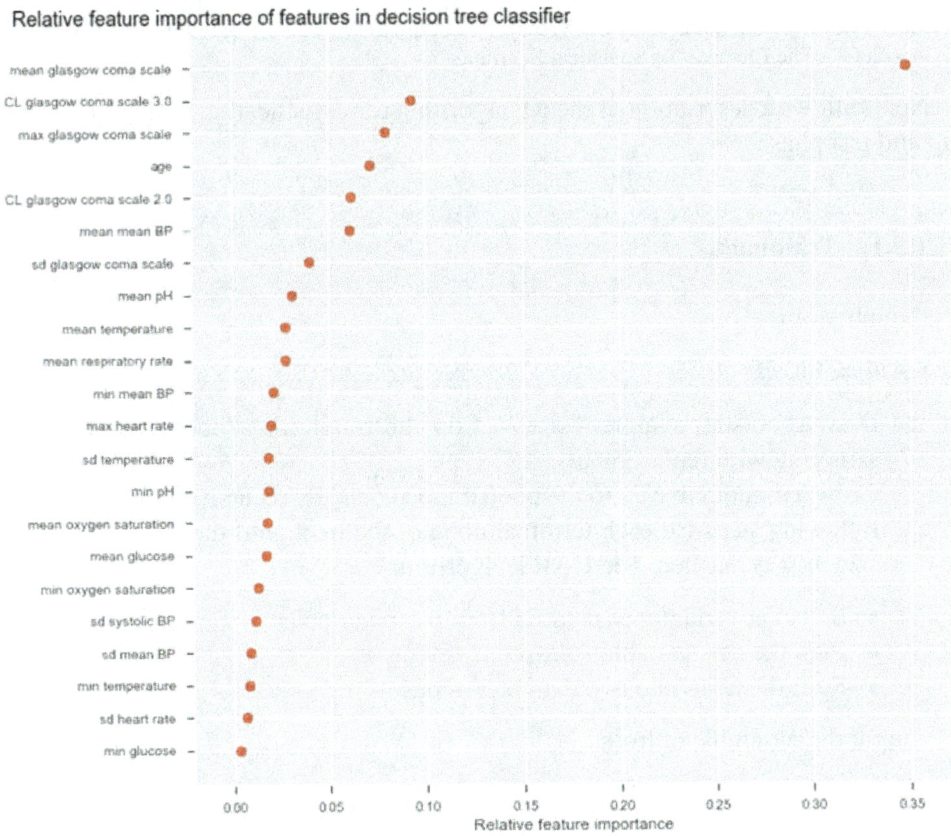

Again, we will store the results, but in this case we need to update the actual number of features used:

```
In [60]: all_results_train =
         all_results_train.append(results_train.rename(index={results_train.index[-1]: 'DT'}))
         all_results_test =
```

```
all_results_test.append(results_test.rename(index={results_test.index[-1]: 'DT'}))
all_results_train.loc['DT', '# features'] = len(pd_list_top)
all_results_test.loc['DT', '# features'] = len(pd_list_top)
```

11.1.5 Ensemble Learning with Random Forest

The rationale behind ensemble learning is the creation of many models such that the combination or selection of their output improves the performance of the overall model. In this chapter we will explore one type of ensemble learning based on decision trees, called random forest.

Random forest (RF) comprises split-variable selection, sub-sampling and bootstrap aggregating (bagging).

> The essential idea in bagging is to average many noisy but approximately unbiased models, and hence reduce the variance. Trees are ideal candidates for bagging, since they can capture complex interaction structures in the data, and if grown sufficiently deep, have relatively low bias. Since trees are notoriously noisy, they benefit greatly from the averaging. Friedman et al. - 2008 - The Elements of Statistical Learning.

Next follows a description of the RF algorithm for classification during the learning and test phases.

11.1.5.1 Training

B : Number of trees

1. For $b = 1$ to B
   1.1. Draw a bootstrap sample of size N_b from the training data (bootstrap = random sampling with replacement).
   1.2. Grow a random tree T_b to the bootstrapped data, by recursively repeating the following steps for each terminal node of the tree, until the minimum node size $n_{\min}$ is reached. See **CART** algorithm.
      - Select m variables at random from the p variables
      - Pick the best variable/split-point among m
      - Split the node into two daughter nodes
2. Output the ensemble of trees

11.1.5.2 Testing

Let $C_b(x_i)$ be the predicted class probability of the bth tree in the ensemble for observation x_i. Then, the predicted class probability of the random forest for observation x_i is:

$$C_{rf}^{B}(x_i) = \frac{1}{B}\sum_{b=1}^{B} C_b(x_i)$$

The predicted class probabilities of an input sample are computed as the mean predicted class probabilities of the trees in the forest. The class probability of a single tree is the fraction of samples of the same class in a leaf.

The algorithm can be implemented in 'sklearn' using the 'RandomForestClassifier'. Similarly to the DT, important parameters to define are:

- **n_estimators**: number of trees in the forest.
- **criterion**: function to measure the quality of a split. Default = 'gini'.
- **max_features**: maximum number of features in each tree. Default is sqrt (n_features).
- **max_depth**: maximum depth of the tree. If None, then nodes are expanded until all leaves are pure or until all leaves contain less than min_samples_split samples.
- **min_samples_split**: minimum number of samples required to split an internal node. Default = 2.
- **min_samples_leaf**: minimum number of samples required to be at a leaf node (external node). Default = 1.
- **random_state**: if int, seed used by the random number generator. Default = None.
- **bootstrap**: Whether bootstrap samples are used when building trees. The subsample size is always the same as the original input sample size but the samples are drawn with replacement if bootstrap = True. Default = True.

The next example shows how to build a RF classifier with 100 trees and a maximum depth of 10:

```
In [61]: from sklearn.ensemble import RandomForestClassifier

         rf = RandomForestClassifier(n_estimators = 100, bootstrap = True, criterion = 'gini',
                                     max_depth = 10, random_state = 2)

         rf.fit(X_train, y_train.values.ravel())
         results_train, results_test, y_pred_prob_train, y_pred_prob_test = model_evaluation(rf,
         X_train, y_train, X_test, y_test, print =1)

         all_results_train =
         all_results_train.append(results_train.rename(index={results_train.index[-1]: 'RF'}))
         all_results_test =
         all_results_test.append(results_test.rename(index={results_test.index[-1]: 'RF'}))
```

```
TRAINING SET
Threshold: 0.4
TP: 818
TN: 1256
FP: 22
FN: 14
Accuracy: 0.98
Sensitivity: 0.98
Specificity: 0.98
AUC: 1.0
```

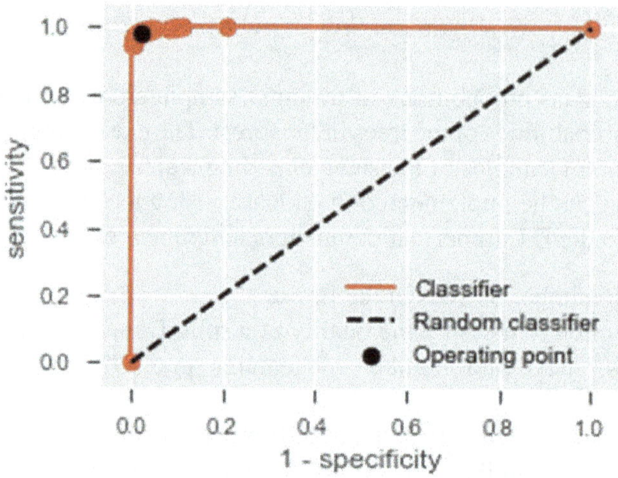


```
TEST SET
Threshold: 0.4
TP: 175
TN: 741
FP: 269
FN: 47
Accuracy: 0.74
Sensitivity: 0.79
Specificity: 0.73
AUC: 0.84
```

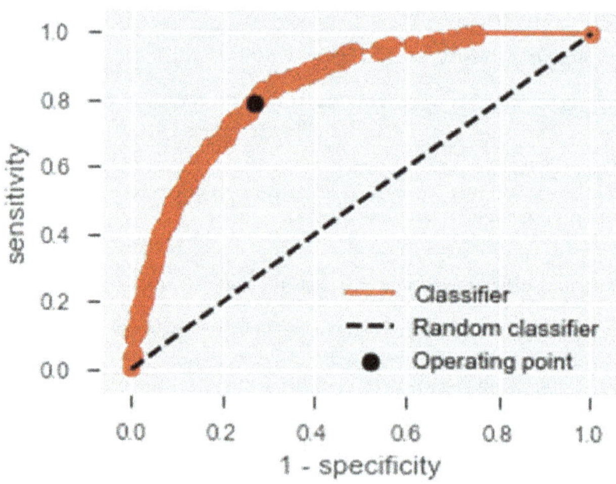

As you can see, in the previous RF configuration the training error is very low. This warrants suspicion of high variance. In fact, the performance in the test set is significantly lower. In order to reduce overfitting, we can reduce the depth of the trees and increase the 'min_samples_split'.

```
In [62]: from sklearn.ensemble import RandomForestClassifier

         print_ = 1
         rf = RandomForestClassifier(n_estimators = 100, bootstrap = True, criterion = 'gini',
                                     max_depth = 7, min_samples_split = 30, random_state = 2)

         rf.fit(X_train, y_train.values.ravel())
         results_train, results_test, y_pred_prob_train, y_pred_prob_test = model_evaluation(rf,
         X_train, y_train, X_test, y_test, print_)

         all_results_train =
         all_results_train.append(results_train.rename(index={results_train.index[-1]: 'RF
         small'}))
         all_results_test =
         all_results_test.append(results_test.rename(index={results_test.index[-1]: 'RF small'}))
```

```
TRAINING SET
Threshold: 0.43
TP: 730
TN: 1120
FP: 158
FN: 102
Accuracy: 0.88
Sensitivity: 0.88
Specificity: 0.88
AUC: 0.95
```

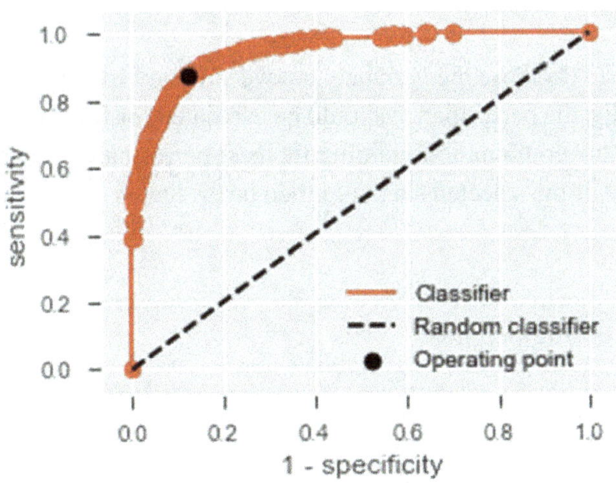

```
TEST SET
Threshold: 0.43
TP: 164
TN: 777
FP: 233
FN: 58
Accuracy: 0.76
Sensitivity: 0.74
Specificity: 0.77
AUC: 0.84
```

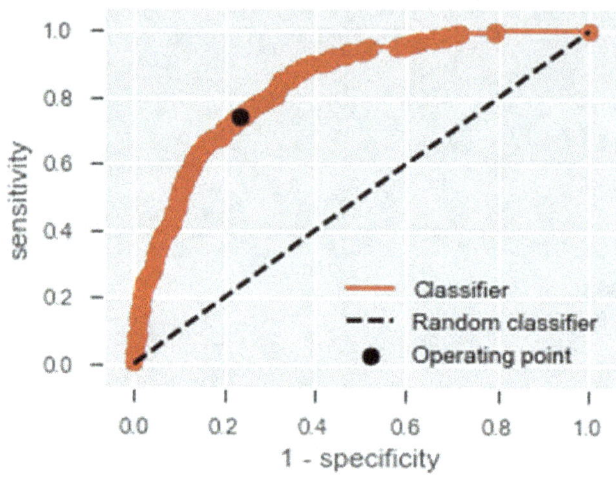

We were able to decrease the variance, but we still have moderate performance in the test set. Ideally, the performance should be evaluated for various combinations of parameters, and the combination yielding the best performance should be selected. The performance of the selected set could then be evaluated using a test set not used before.

11.1.5.3 Feature Importance

At each split in each tree, the improvement in the split-criterion (G) is the importance measure attributed to the splitting feature and is accumulated over all the trees in the forest separately for each feature. The same function created for DT can be used for RF:

```
In [63]: pd_list_top = plot_feat_importance(X_train.columns, rf.feature_importances_, 40)
```

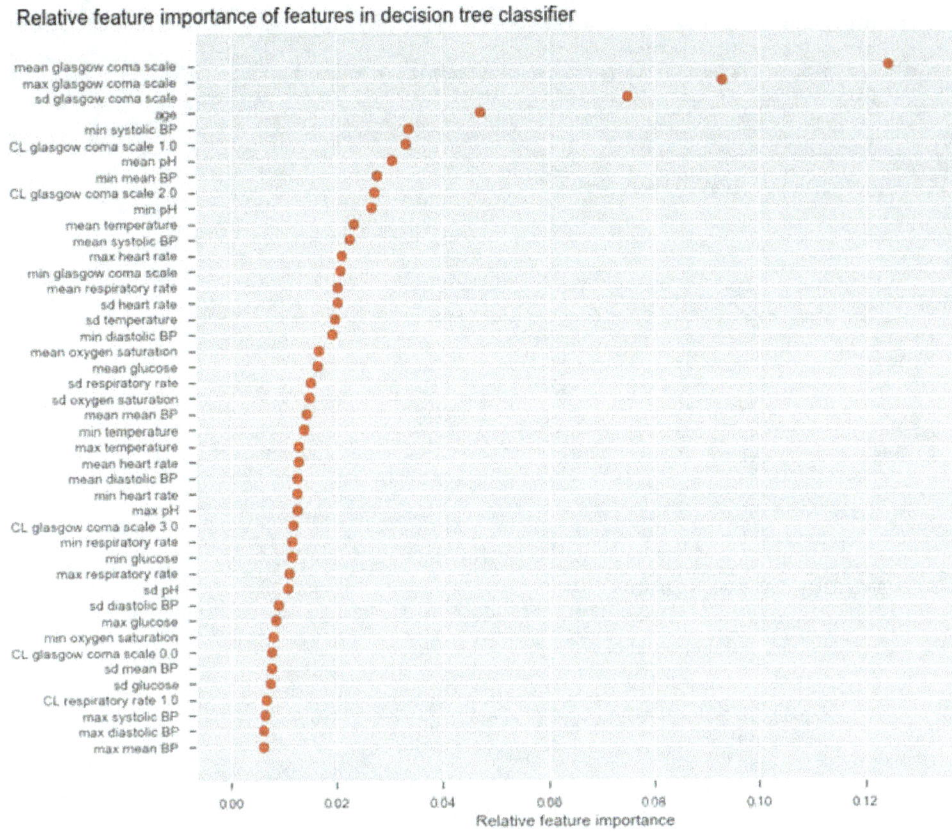

Update the actual number of features used in the RF:

```
In [64]: all_results_train.loc['RF small', '# features'] = len(pd_list_top)
         all_results_test.loc['RF small', '# features'] = len(pd_list_top)
```

The features to which RF assigns higher feature importance are consistent with previous findings. Several features extracted from GCS appear at the top.

11.1.6 Comparison of Classifiers

The next example summarizes the performance of several classifiers and their ability to generalize. To better assess the classifiers ability to generalize, the difference between training and test performance is plotted.

```
In [65]: print('Performance in training set')
         display.display(np.round(all_results_train, decimals = 2))
         print()

         print('Performance in test set')
         display.display(np.round(all_results_test, decimals = 2))
         print()

         diff = all_results_train-all_results_test
         diff[['AUC', 'Sensitivity','Specificity']].plot(kind = 'bar', figsize = (10,3))
```

```
plt.ylabel('Difference in performance')
plt.xticks(rotation=None)
plt.title('Difference in performance (training - test)')
plt.show()
```

```
Performance in training set
```

	Threshold	AUC	Sensitivity	Specificity	# features
LR SFS	0.39	0.82	0.76	0.76	11.0
LR RFE	0.40	0.85	0.77	0.77	13.0
KNN SFS	NaN	NaN	NaN	NaN	NaN
DT	0.44	0.87	0.82	0.77	22.0
RF	0.40	1.00	0.98	0.98	85.0
RF small	0.43	0.95	0.88	0.88	44.0

```
Performance in test set
```

	Threshold	AUC	Sensitivity	Specificity	# features
LR SFS	0.39	0.79	0.71	0.72	11.0
LR RFE	0.40	0.82	0.73	0.74	13.0
KNN SFS	1.00	0.69	0.56	0.81	11.0
DT	0.44	0.77	0.72	0.70	22.0
RF	0.40	0.84	0.79	0.73	85.0
RF small	0.43	0.84	0.74	0.77	44.0

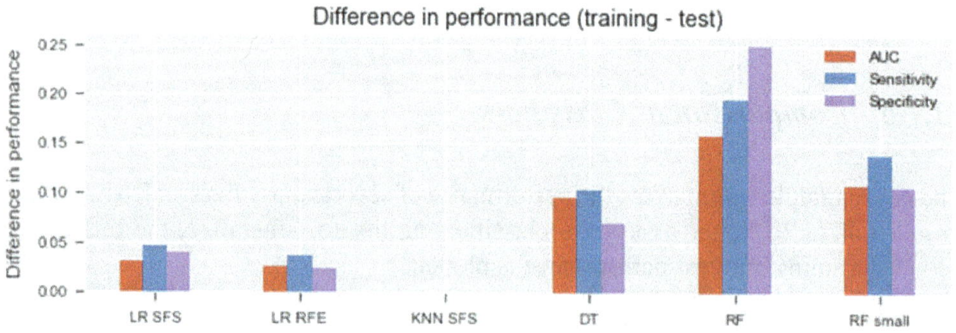

11.2 Limitations

In the next section, critical aspects of the study conducted are discussed.

11.2.1 Selecting One Model

What is the best model? At this point it is probable that the reader is posing this question. The answer to what is the best model, or what model should be selected, is not straightforward. At this point, it really is about selecting a good path to continue exploring. A single decision tree is clearly not the way to go in terms of performance, but it can be useful if interpretability is a must. LR is also interpretable when the feature set contains a resonable number of features. So if interpretability is important, LF with RFE or SFS should be considered. RF performs well in the test set but the increase in performance relative to simpler models is very small. The choice depends on reaching a good trade-off between what's more important; e.g., if sensitivity is very important, and not so much interpretability, then the first RF should be chosen.

11.2.2 Training, Testing and Validation

Before making any conclusions about performance, it is advisable to change the data partitions used for training, testing and validating. A single data partitioning has been used in order to facilitate the presentation of ideas, but ideally the evaluation should not be limited to a single random data division. Cross validation can be used to investigate the variablity in performance when different data partitions are used. Following this approach, all data is used for training and testing the models and the results are averaged over the rounds.

11.2.3 Bias/variance

Decision tree based models have high variance, i.e., the trees are probably overfitting the training data and this hampers their ability to generalize. Again, cross-validation should be performed—we would likely get very different DTs for different training partitions (which is why RF is better!). As mentioned before, the bias/variance problem could be addressed by training/validating models for a range of distinct combinations of parameters and selecting a set that minimizes overfitting to the training data (low bias) and that at the same time performs well in the validation set (low variance).

11.3 Conclusions

This chapter provides a step by step illustrative guideline of how to conduct a machine learning project for healthcare research and the tools needed to easily implement it using the Python programming language and Jupyter notebook documents. It focuses on exploratory data analysis, variable selection, data preprocessing, data analysis, feature construction, feature selection, performance evaluation and model training and testing. The steps conducted before machine learning should allow the researcher to better understand how the data can be prepared for modeling. Tools for data analysis have also been presented in order to guide decisions and point towards interesting research directions. At each step, decisions are made based on the requisites of the problem. It should be emphasized however that a single answer to how to best conduct a project similar to the one presented here does not exist. In particular, many decisions were made in order to preserve simplicity and improve model interpretability, for example when deciding to extract summary statistics and snapshots measurements from the time series without resorting to more complex approaches that could have led to better performance.

11.4 Exercises

11.4.1 Daily Prediction

It is useful to evaluate the performance of the classifier using data from the first day. It will give us a more realistic sense of how the classifier would behave in a real setting if we wanted a decision at the end of the first day.

We have performed dimensionality reduction by extracting relevant information from the complete time series (48 h). Investigate how the performance changes if you do this separately for each 24 h.

11.4.2 Clustering Patterns

Clustering has been employed for patient stratification. Data were normalized for each patient individually so that the groups would reflect physiological time trends. How do the patterns change if:

1. the random seed used to generate the training and test sets changes;
2. the random seed used to initiate the cluster centers changes;
3. data is not normalized;
4. data is normalized for the entire training set at once?

11.4.3 Class Imbalance

Undersampling has been used in order to mitigate bias toward a predominant class. Class balancing can also be performed by sampling an equal number of observations from each class. In 'sklearn', you can use the parameter 'class_weight' in order to control for imbalanced training data when learning logistic regression, decision trees or random forest:

- class_weight = {class_label: weight}: weights associated with classes. If not given, all classes are assumed to have weight one.
- class_weight = 'balanced': uses the values of y to automatically adjust weights inversely proportional to class frequencies in the input data.

Investigate how class_weight = 'balanced' impacts the performance of the models.

11.4.4 Bias/Variance

Investigate how bias and variance are affected by different choices of parameters.

11.5 Recommended Literature

1. Machine Learning Yearning (2018) by Andre Ng (draft version currently available)
2. The elements of statistical learning (2001) by Friedman J, Hastie T, Tibshirani R.
3. Secondary Analysis of Electronic Health Records (2016) by MIT Critical Data
4. Python Data Science Handbook (2016) by Jake VanderPlas
5. Hands-On Machine Learning with Scikit-Learn and TensorFlow (2017) by Aurélien Géron

Acknowledgements This work was supported by the Portuguese Foundation for Science & Technology, through IDMEC, under LAETA, project UID/EMS/50022/2019 and LISBOA-01-0145-FEDER-031474 supported by Programa Operational Regional de Lisboa by FEDER and FCT.

12

Machine Learning Techniques and their Application in Clinical Prediction Tasks

Wei-Hung Weng

Abstract In this chapter, we provide a brief overview of applying machine learning techniques for clinical prediction tasks. We begin with a quick introduction to the concepts of machine learning, and outline some of the most common machine learning algorithms. Next, we demonstrate how to apply the algorithms with appropriate toolkits to conduct machine learning experiments for clinical prediction tasks. This chapter is composed of five sections. First, we will explain why machine learning techniques are helpful for researchers in solving clinical prediction problems (Sect. 12.1). Understanding the motivations behind machine learning approaches in healthcare are essential, since precision and accuracy are often critical in healthcare problems, and everything from diagnostic decisions to predictive clinical analytics could dramatically benefit from data-based processes with improved efficiency and reliability. In the second section, we will introduce several important concepts in machine learning in a colloquial manner, such as learning scenarios, objective/target function, error and loss function and metrics, optimization and model validation, and finally a summary of model selection methods (Sect. 12.2). These topics will help us utilize machine learning algorithms in an appropriate way. Following that, we will introduce some popular machine learning algorithms for prediction problems (Sect. 12.3), for example, logistic regression, decision tree and support vector machine. Then, we will discuss some limitations and pitfalls of using the machine learning approach (Sect. 12.4). Lastly, we will provide case studies using real intensive care unit (ICU) data from a publicly available dataset, PhysioNet Challenge 2012, as well as the breast tumor data from Breast Cancer Wisconsin (Diagnostic) Database, and summarize what we have presented in this chapter (Sect. 12.5).

Keywords Machine Learning · Artificial Intelligence · Healthcare · Clinical Data Medical Computing

W. H. Weng (✉)
CSAIL, MIT, Cambridge, MA, USA
e-mail: ckbjimmy@mit.edu

Learning Objectives

- Understand the basics of machine learning techniques and the reasons behind why they are useful for solving clinical prediction problems.
- Understand the intuition behind some machine learning models, including regression, decision trees, and support vector machines.
- Understand how to apply these models to clinical prediction problems using publicly available datasets via case studies.

12.1 Why Machine Learning?

Machine learning is an interdisciplinary field which consists of computer science, mathematics, and statistics. It is also an approach toward building intelligent machines for artificial intelligence (AI). Different from rule-based symbolic AI, the idea of utilizing machine learning for AI is to learn from data (examples and experiences). Instead of explicitly programming hand-crafted rules, we construct a model for prediction by feeding data into a machine learning algorithm, and the algorithm will learn an optimized function based on the data and the specific task. Such data-driven methodology is now the state-of-the-art approach of various research domains, such as computer vision (Krizhevsky et al. 2012), natural language processing (NLP) (Yala et al. 2017), and speech-to-text translation (Wu et al. 2016; Chung et al. 2018, 2019), for many complex real-world applications.

Due to the increased popularity of the electronic health record (EHR) system in recent years, massive quantities of healthcare data have been generated (Henry et al. 2016). Machine learning for healthcare therefore becomes an emerging applied domain. Recently, researchers and clinicians have started applying machine learning algorithms to solve the problems of clinical outcome prediction (Ghassemi et al. 2014), diagnosis (Gulshan et al. 2016; Esteva et al. 2017; Liu et al. 2017; Chung and Weng 2017; Nagpal et al. 2018), treatment and optimal decision making (Raghu et al. 2017; Weng et al. 2017; Komorowski et al. 2018) using data in different modalities, such as structured lab measurements (Pivovarov et al. 2015), claims data (Doshi-Velez et al. 2014; Pivovarov et al. 2015; Choi et al. 2016), free texts (Pivovarov et al. 2015; Weng et al. 2018, 2019), images (Gulshan et al. 2016; Esteva et al. 2017; Bejnordi 2017; Chen et al. 2018), physiological signals (Lehman et al. 2018), and even cross-modal information (Hsu et al. 2018; Liu et al. 2019).

Instead of traditional ad-hoc healthcare data analytics, which usually requires expert-intensive efforts for collecting data and designing limited hand-crafted features, machine learning-based approaches help us recognize patterns inside the data and allow us to perform personalized clinical prediction with more generalizable models (Gehrmann et al. 2018). They help us maximize the utilization of massive but complex EHR data. In this chapter, we will focus on how to tackle clinical prediction problems using a machine learning-based approach.

12.2 General Concepts of Learning

12.2.1 Learning Scenario for Clinical Prediction

We start with how to frame your clinical problem into a machine learning prediction problem with a simple example. Assuming that you want to build a model for predicting the mortality of ICU patients with continuous renal replacement therapy and you have a large ICU database, which includes hundreds of variables such as vital signs, lab data, demographics, medications, and even clinical notes and reports, the clinical problem can be reframed as a task: "Given data with hundreds of input variables, I want to learn a model from the data that can correctly make a prediction given a new datapoint." That is, the output of the function (model) should be as close as possible to the outcome of what exactly happened (the ground truth). Machine learning algorithm is here to help to find the best function from a set of functions. This is a typical machine learning scenario, which is termed supervised learning. In such a case, you may do the following steps:

- Define the outcome of your task
- Consult with domain experts to identify important features/variables
- Select an appropriate algorithm (or design a new machine learning algorithm) with a suitable parameter selection
- Find an optimized model with a subset of data (training data) with the algorithm
- Evaluate the model with another subset of data (testing data) with appropriate metrics
- Deploy the prediction model on real-world data.

At the end of the chapter, we will show an exercise notebook that will help you go through the concepts mentioned above.

12.2.2 Machine Learning Scenarios

There are many machine learning scenarios, such as supervised learning, unsupervised learning, semi-supervised learning, reinforcement learning, and transfer learning. We will only focus on the first two main categories, supervised learning and unsupervised learning. Both of the scenarios learn from the underlying data distribution, or to put it simply, find patterns inside data. The difference between them is that you have annotated data under the supervised scenario but only unlabelled data under unsupervised learning scenario.

12.2.2.1 Supervised Learning

Supervised learning is the most common scenario for practical machine learning tasks if the outcome is well-defined, for example, if you are predicting patient mortality, hospital length of stay, or drug response. In general, the supervised learning algorithm will try to learn how to build a classifier for predicting the outcome variable y given input x, which is a mapping function f where $y = f(x)$. The classifier will be built by an algorithm along with a set of data $\{x_1, ..., x_n\}$ with the corresponding outcome label $\{y_1, ..., y_n\}$. Supervised learning can be categorized by two criteria, either by type of prediction or by type of model. First, it can be separated into regression or classification problems. For predicting continuous outcomes, using regression methods such as linear regression is suitable. For class prediction, classification algorithms such as logistic regression, naive Bayes, decision trees or support vector machines (SVM) (Cortes and Vapnik 1995) will be a better choice. For example, linear regression is suitable for children height prediction problem whereas SVM is better for binary mortality prediction.

Regarding the goal of the learning process, a discriminative model such as regression, trees and SVMs can learn the decision boundary within the data. However, a generative model like naive Bayes will learn the probability distributions of the data.

12.2.2.2 Unsupervised Learning

Without corresponding output variables (y), the unsupervised learning algorithms discover latent structures and patterns directly from the given unlabeled data $\{x_1, ..., x_n\}$.

There is no ground truth in the unsupervised learning, therefore, the machine will only find associations or clusters inside the data. For example, we may discover hidden subtypes in a disease using an unsupervised approach (Ghassemi et al. 2014).

12.2.2.3 Other Scenario

Other scenarios such as reinforcement learning (RL) frame a decision making problem into a computer agent interaction with a dynamic environment (Silver et al. 2016), in which the agent attempts to reach the best reward based on feedback when it navigates the state and action space. Using a clinical scenario as an example, the agent (the RL algorithm) will try to improve the model parameters based on iteratively simulating the state (patient condition) and action (giving fluid or vasopressor for hypotension), obtain the feedback reward (mortality or not), and eventually converge to a model that may yield optimal decisions (Raghu et al. 2017).

12.2.3 Find the Best Function

To estimate and find the best mapping function in the above scenarios, the process of optimization is needed. However, we do need to define some criteria to tell us how well the function (model) can predict the task. Therefore, we need a loss function and a cost function (objective function) for this purpose.

Loss function defines the difference between the output of model y and the real data value $\hat{y}$. Different machine learning algorithms may use different loss functions, for example, least squared error for linear regression, logistic loss for logistic regression, and hinge loss for SVM (Table 12.1). Cost function is the summation of loss functions of each training data point. Using loss functions, we can define the cost function to evaluate model performance. Through loss and cost functions, we can compute the performance of functions on the whole dataset.

In unsupervised learning setting, the algorithms have no real data value to compute the loss function. In such case, we can use the input itself as the output and compute the difference between input and output. For example, we use reconstruction loss for autoencoder, a kind of unsupervised learning algorithms, to evaluate whether the model can reconstruct the input from hidden states inside the model.

There is a mathematical proof for this learning problem to explain why machine learning is feasible even if the function space is infinite. Since our goal is not to explain the mathematics and mechanism of machine learning, further details on why there is a finite bound on the generalization error are not mentioned here. For readers who are interested in the theory of machine learning, such as Hoeffding's inequality that gives a probability upper bound, Vapnik–Chervonenkis (VC) dimension and VC generalization bound, please refer to other textbooks (Abu-Mostafa et al. 2012).

12.2.4 Metrics

Choosing an appropriate numeric evaluation metric for optimization is crucial. Different evaluation metrics are applied to different scenarios and problems.

Table 12.1 Examples of commonly-used loss functions in machine learning

Task	Error type	Loss function	Note
Regression	Mean-squared error	$\frac{1}{n}\sum_{i=1}^{n}(y_i-\hat{y}_i)^2$	Easy to learn but sensitive to outliers (MSE, L2 loss)
	Mean absolute error	$\frac{1}{n}\sum_{i=1}^{n}\lvert y_i-\hat{y}_i\rvert$	Robust to outliers but not differentiable (MAE, L1 loss)
Classification	Cross entropy = Log loss	$-\frac{1}{n}\sum_{i=1}^{n}[y_i\log(\hat{y}_i)+(1-y_i)\log(1-\hat{y}_i)]=-\frac{1}{n}\sum_{i=1}^{n}p_i\log q_i$	Quantify the difference between two probability distributions
	Hinge loss	$\frac{1}{n}\sum_{i=1}^{n}max(0,1-y_i\hat{y}_i)$	For support vector machine
	KL divergence	$D_{KL}(p\|\|q)=\sum_i p_i(\log\frac{p_i}{q_i})$	Quantify the difference between two probability distributions

12.2.4.1 Supervised Learning

In classification problems, accuracy, precision/positive predictive value (PPV), recall/sensitivity, specificity, and the F1 score are usually used. We use a confusion matrix to show the relation between these metrics (Table 12.2).

The area under receiver operating curve (AUROC) is a very common metric, which sums up the area under the curve in the plot with x-axis of false positive rate (FPR, also known as 1-specificity), and y-axis of true positive rate (TPR) (Fig. 12.1). FPR and TPR values may change based on the threshold of your subjective choice.

In a regression problem, the adjusted R-squared value is commonly used for evaluation. The R-squared value, also known as the coefficient of determination, follows the equation and is defined by the total sum of squares (SStot) and the residual sum of squares (SSres). The detailed equations are as follows:

Table 12.2 Commonly-used metrics in machine learning

		Predicted		
		True	False	
Actual	True	True positive (TP)	False negative (FN) Type II error	Recall = Sensitivity = $\frac{TP}{TP+FN}$
	False	False positive (FP) Type I error	True negative (TN)	Specificity = $\frac{TN}{TN+FP}$
		Precision = $\frac{TP}{TP+FP}$		Accuracy = $\frac{TP+TN}{TP+TN+FP+FN}$ F1 = $\frac{2\times Precision \times Recall}{Precision+Recall}$

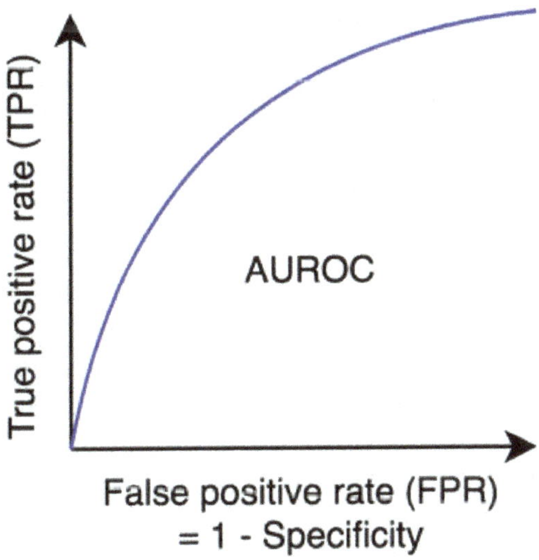

Fig. 12.1 Example of AUROC

$$R^2 = 1 - \frac{SS_{res}}{SS_{tot}} = 1 - \frac{\sum_{i=1}^{m}(y_i - f(x_i))^2}{\sum_{i=1}^{m}(y_i - \hat{y}_i)^2}$$

$$\text{Adjusted } R^2 = 1 - \frac{(1 - R^2)(m - 1)}{m - n - 1}$$

There are also other metrics for regression, such as Akaike information criterion (AIC) and Bayesian information criterion (BIC), for different study purposes.

12.2.4.2 Unsupervised Learning

Since there are no ground truth labels for unsupervised scenarios, evaluation metrics of unsupervised learning settings are relatively difficult to define and usually depend on the algorithms in question. For example, the Calinski-Harabaz index and silhouette coefficient have been used to evaluate *k*-means clustering. Reconstruction error is used for autoencoder, a kind of neural network architecture for learning data representation.

12.2.5 Model Validation

The next step after deciding the algorithm is to get your data ready for training a model for your task. In practice, we split the whole dataset into three pieces:

- Training set for model training. You will run the selected machine learning algorithm only on this subset.
- Development (a.k.a. dev, validation) set, also called hold-out, for parameter tuning and feature selection. This subset is only for optimization and model validation.
- Testing set for evaluating model performance. We only apply the model for prediction here, but won't change any content in the model at this moment.

There are a few things that we need to keep in mind:

- It is better to have your training, dev and testing sets all from the same data distribution instead of having them too different (e.g. training/dev on male patients but testing on female patients), otherwise you may face the problem of overfitting, in which your model will fit the data too well in training or dev sets but find it difficult to generalize to the test data. In this situation, the trained model will not be able to be applied to other cases.
- It is important to prevent using any data in the dev set or testing set for model training. Test data leakage, i.e. having part of testing data from training data, may cause the overfitting of the model to your test data and erroneously gives you a high performance but a bad model.

There is no consensus on the relative proportions of the three subsets. However, people usually allocate 20–30% of the whole dataset for their testing set. The proportion can be smaller if you have more data.

12.2.5.1 Cross-Validation

The other commonly used approach for model validation is k-fold cross validation (CV). The goal of k-fold CV is to reduce the overfitting of the initial training set by further training several models with the same algorithm but with different training/dev set splitting.

In k-fold CV, we split the whole dataset into k folds and train the model k times. In each training, we iteratively leave one different fold out for validation, and train on the remaining $k - 1$ folds. The final error is the average of errors over k times of training (Fig. 12.2). In practice, we usually use $k = 5$ or 10. The extreme case for n cases is n-fold CV, which is also called leave-one-out CV (LOOCV).

Please keep in mind that the testing set is completely excluded from the process of CV. Only training and dev sets are involved in this process.

12.2.6 *Diagnostics*

After the first iteration of model training and evaluation, you may find that the trained model does not perform well on the unseen testing data. To address the issue of error in machine learning, we need to conduct some diagnostics regarding bias and variance in the model in order to achieve a model with low bias and low variance.

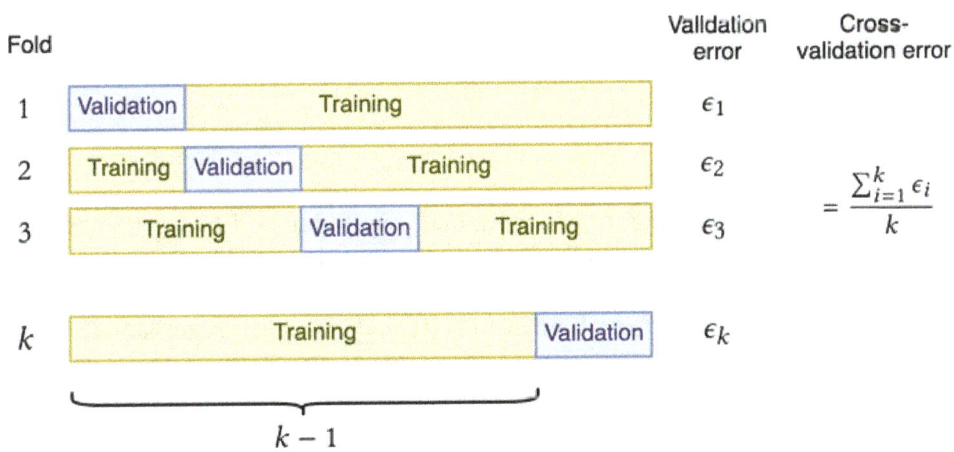

Fig. 12.2 K-fold cross-validation

Table 12.3 The characteristic of high bias and high variance

	Training error	Validation error	Approach
High bias	High	Low	Increase complexity
High variance	Low	High	Decrease complexity Add more data

12.2.6.1 Bias and Variance

The bias of a model is the difference between the prediction model and the correct model for given data points. That is, it is the algorithm's error rate on the training set. This is an underfitting problem, whereby the model can't capture the trend of the data well due to an excessively simple model. One potential solution is to make the model more complex, which can be done by reducing regularization (Sect. 12.2.6.2), or configuring and adding more input features, for example, stacking more layers if you are using a deep learning approach. However, it is possible that the outcome of complex model is high variance.

The variance of a model is the variability of the model prediction for given data points. It is the model error rate difference between training and dev sets. Problems of high variance are usually related to the issue of overfitting. i.e. hard to generalize to unseen data. The possible solution is to simplify the model, such as using regularization, reducing the number of features, or add more training data. Yet the simpler model may also suffer from the issue of high bias.

High bias and high variance can happen simultaneously with very bad models. To achieve the optimal error rate, a.k.a. Bayes error rate, which is an unavoidable bias from the most optimized model, we need to do iterative experiments to find the optimal bias and variance tradeoff.

Finally, a good practice of investigating bias and variance is to plot the informative learning curve with training and validation errors. In Fig. 12.3 and Table 12.3 we demonstrate a few cases of diagnostics as examples.

12.2.6.2 Regularization

The goal of regularization is to prevent model overfitting and high variance. The most common regularization techniques include Least absolute shrinkage and selection operator (LASSO regression, L1-regularization) (Tibshirani 1996), ridge regression (L2-regression) (Hoerl and Kennard 1970), and elastic net regression (a linear combination of L1 and L2 regularization) (Zou and Hastie 2005).

In practice, we add a weighted penalty term λ to the cost function. For L1-regularization, we add the absolute value of the magnitude of coefficient as penalty term, and in L2-regularization we add the squared value of magnitude instead (Table 12.4).

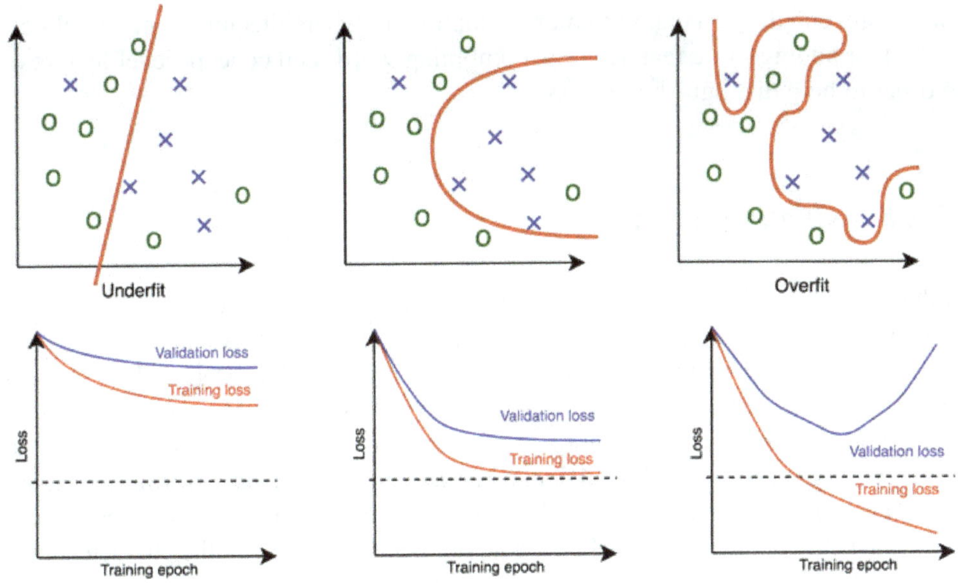

Fig. 12.3 Bias and variance

Table 12.4 L1 and L2-regularized logistic regression

Regularization	Equation
L1 (LASSO)	$\sum_{i=1}^{m}(y_i - \sum_{j=1}^{n}\beta_j x_{ij})^2 + \lambda\sum_{j=1}^{n}\lvert\beta_j\rvert$
L2 (Ridge)	$\sum_{i=1}^{m}(y_i - \sum_{j=1}^{n}\beta_j x_{ij})^2 + \lambda\sum_{j=1}^{n}\beta_j^2$

L1-regularization is also a good technique for feature selection since it can "shrink" the coefficients of less important features to zero and remove them. In contrast, L2-regularization just makes the coefficients smaller, but not to zero.

12.2.7 Error Analysis

It is an important practice to construct your first prediction pipeline as soon as possible and iteratively improve its performance by error analysis. Error analysis is a critical step to examine the performance between your model and the optimized one. To do the analysis, it is necessary to manually go through some erroneously predicted data from the dev set.

The error analysis can help you understand potential problems in the current algorithm setting. For example, the misclassified cases usually come from specific classes (e.g. patients with cardiovascular issues might get confused with those with renal problems since there are some shared pathological features between two organ systems) or inputs with specific conditions (Weng et al. 2017). Such misclassification can be prevented by changing to more complex model architecture (e.g. neural networks), or adding more features (e.g. combining word- and concept-level features), in order to help distinguish the classes.

12.2.8 Ablation Analysis

Ablation analysis is a critical step for identifying important factors in the model. Once you obtain an ideal model, it is necessary to compare it with some simple but robust models, such as linear or logistic regression model. This step is also essential for research projects, since the readers of your work will want to know what factors and methods are related to the improvement of model performance. For example, the deep learning approach of clinical document deidentification outperforms traditional natural language processing approach. In the paper using neural network for deidentification (Dernoncourt et al. 2017), the authors demonstrate that the character-level token embedding technique had the greatest effect on model performance, and this became the critical factor of their study.

12.3 Learning Algorithms

In this section, we briefly introduce the concepts of some algorithm families that can be used in the clinical prediction tasks. For supervised learning, we will discuss linear models, tree-based models and SVM. For unsupervised learning, we will discuss the concepts of clustering and dimensionality reduction algorithms. We will skip the neural network method in this chapter. Please refer to programming tutorial part 3 or a deep learning textbook for further information (Goodfellow et al. 2016).

12.3.1 Supervised Learning

12.3.1.1 Linear Models

Linear models are commonly used not only in machine learning but also in statistical analysis. They are widely adopted in the clinical world and can usually be provided as baseline models for clinical machine learning tasks. In this class of algorithms, we usually use linear regression for regression problems and logistic regression for classification problems.

The pros of linear models include their interpretability, less computational cost as well as less complexity comparing to other classical machine learning algorithms. The downside is their inferior performance. However, these are common trade-off features in model selection. It is still worthwhile to start from this simple but powerful family of algorithms.

12.3.1.2 Tree-Based Models

Tree-based models can be used for both regression and classification problems. Decision tree, also known as classification and regression trees (CART), is one of the most common tree-based models (Breiman 2017). It follows the steps below to find the best tree:

- It looks across all possible thresholds across all possible features and picks the single feature split that best separates the data
- The data is split on that feature at a specific threshold that yields the highest performance
- It iteratively repeats the above two steps until reaching the maximal tree depth, or until all the leaves are pure.

There are many parameters that should be considered while using the decision tree algorithm. The following are some important parameters:

- Splitting criteria: by Gini index or entropy
- Tree size: tree depth, tree pruning
- Number of samples: minimal samples in a leaf, or minimal sample to split a node.

The biggest advantage of a decision tree is providing model interpretability and actionable decision. Since the tree is represented in a binary way, the trained tree model can be easily converted into a set of rules. For example, in their paper, Fonarow and colleagues utilized CART to create a series of clinical rules (Fonarow et al. 2005). However, decision trees may have high variance and yield an inferior performance.

Random forest is another tree-based algorithm that combines the idea of bagging and subsampling features (Breiman 2001). In brief, it tries to ensemble the results and performances of a number of decision trees that were built by randomly selected sets of features. The algorithm can be explained as follows:

- Pick a random subset of features
- Create a bootstrap sample of data (randomly resample the data)
- Build a decision tree on this data
- Iteratively perform the above steps until termination.

Random forest is a robust classifier that usually works well on most of the supervised learning problems, but a main concern is model interpretability. There are also other tree-based models such as adaptive boosting (Adaboost) and gradient boosting algorithms, which attempt to combine multiple weaker learners into a stronger model (Freund et al. 1999; Friedman 2001).

12.3.1.3 Support Vector Machine (SVM)

SVM is a very powerful family of machine learning algorithms (Cortes and Vapnik 1995). The goal of SVM is to attempt to find a hyperplane (e.g. a line in 2D, a plane in 3D, or a n-dimension structure in a $n + 1$ dimensions space) to separate data points into two sides, and to maximize the minimal distance of the hyperplane from the sentinel data points (Fig. 12.4).

SVM also works for non-linear separable data. It uses a technique called "kernel trick" that linearly splits the data in another vector space, then converts the space back to the original one later (Fig. 12.5). The commonly used kernels include linear kernel, radial basis function (RBF) kernel and polynomial kernel.

Regarding the optimization, we use hinge loss to train SVM. The pros of using SVM is its superior performance, yet the model's inferior interpretability limits its applications in the healthcare domain.

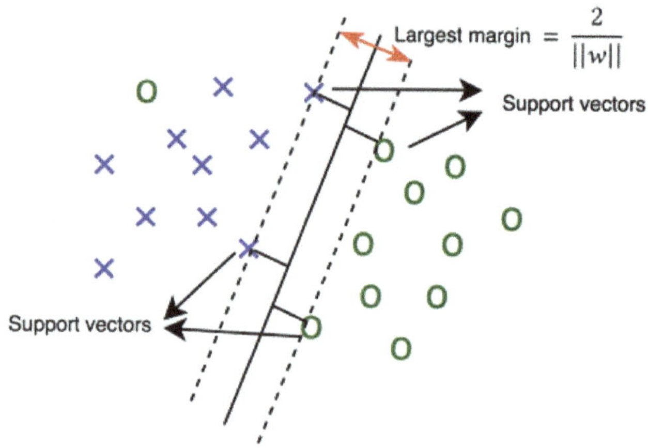

Fig. 12.4 Hyperplane of SVM to linearly separate samples

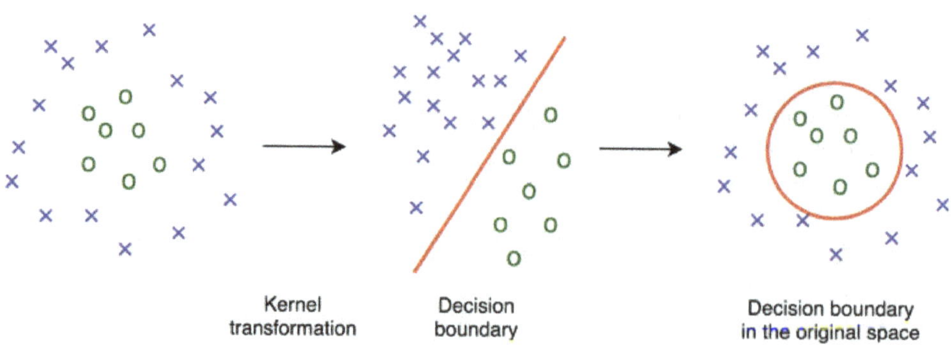

Fig. 12.5 Kernel trick of SVM

12.3.2 *Unsupervised Learning*

In the previous section, we mentioned that the goal of unsupervised learning is to discover hidden patterns inside data. We can use clustering algorithms to aggregate data points into several clusters and investigate the characteristics of each cluster. We can also use dimensionality reduction algorithms to transform a high-dimensional into a smaller-dimensional vector space for further machine learning steps.

12.3.2.1 Clustering

K-means clustering, Expectation-Maximization (EM) algorithm, hierarchical clustering are all common clustering methods. In this section, we will just introduce k-means clustering. The goal of k-means clustering is to find latent groups in the data, with the number of groups represented by the variable k.

The simplified steps of k-means clustering are (Fig. 12.6):

- Randomly initializing k points as the centroids of the k clusters
- Assigning data points to the nearest centroid and forming clusters
- Recomputing and updating centroids based on the mean value of data points in the cluster
- Repeating step 2 and 3 until there is convergence.

The k-means algorithm is guaranteed to converge to a final result. However, this converged state may be local optimum and therefore there is a need to experiment several times to explore the variability of results.

The obtained final k centroids, as well as the cluster labels of data points, can all serve as new features for further machine learning tasks, as shown in Sect. 9 of the "Applied Statistical Learning in Python" chapter. Regarding choosing the cluster number k, there are several techniques for k value validation. The most common

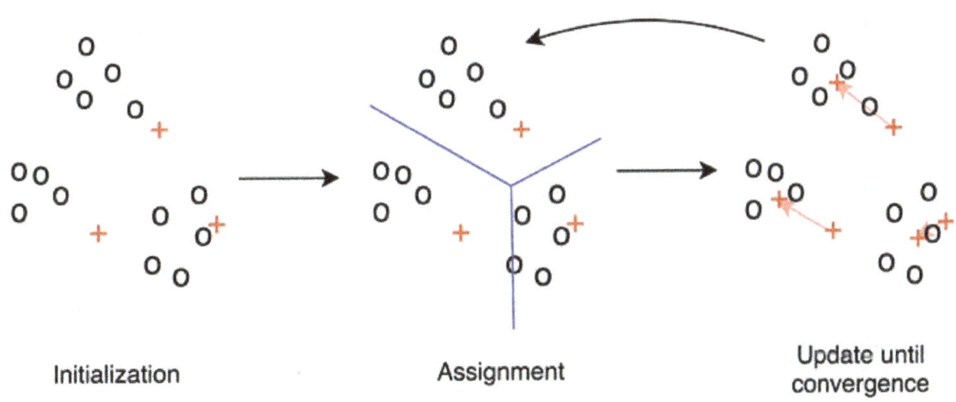

Fig. 12.6 Steps of k-means clustering

methods include the elbow method, silhouette coefficient, or the Calinski-Harabaz index. However, it is very useful to decide *k* if you already have some clinical domain insights about potential cluster number.

12.3.2.2 Dimensionality Reduction

While dealing with clinical data, it is possible that you are faced with a very high-dimensional but sparse dataset. Such characteristics may decrease the model performance even if you use machine algorithms such as SVM, random forest or even deep learning due to the risk of overfitting. A potential solution is to utilize dimensionality reduction algorithms to convert the dataset into lower dimensional vector space. Principal component analysis (PCA) is a method that finds the principal components of the data by transforming data points into a new coordinate system (Jolliffe et al. 2011). The first axis of the new coordinate system corresponds to the first principal component (PC1), which explains the most variance in the data and can serve as the most important feature of the dataset.

PCA is a linear algorithm and therefore it is hard to interpret the complex polynomial relationship between features. Also, PCA may not be able to represent similar data points of high-dimensional data that are close together since the linear algorithm does not consider non-linear manifolds.

The non-linear dimensionality reduction algorithm, t-Distributed Stochastic Neighbor Embedding (t-SNE), becomes an alternative when we want to explore or visualize the high-dimensional data (van der Maaten and Hinton 2008). t-SNE considers probability distributions with random walk on neighborhood graphs on the curved manifold to find the patterns of data. Autoencoder is another dimensionality reduction algorithm based on a neural network architecture for learning data representation by minimizing the difference between the input and output of the network (Rumelhart et al. 1988; Hinton et al. 2006).

The dimensionality reduction algorithms are good at representing multi-dimensional data. Also, a smaller set of features learned from dimensionality reduction algorithms may not only reduce the complexity of the model, but also decrease model training time, as well as inference (classification/prediction) time.

12.4 Programming Exercise

We provide three tutorials for readers to have some hands-on exercises of learning basic machine learning concepts, algorithms and toolkits for clinical prediction tasks. They can be accessed through Google colab and Python Jupyter notebook with two real-world datasets:

- Breast Cancer Wisconsin (Diagnostic) Database
- Preprocessed ICU data from PhysioNet Challenge 2012 Database.

The learning objectives of these tutorial include:

- Learn how to use Google colab/Jupyter notebook
- Learn how to build and diagnose machine learning models for clinical classification and clustering tasks.

In part 1, we will go through the basics of machine learning concepts through classification problems. In part 2, we will go deeper into unsupervised learning methods for clustering and visualization. In part 3, we will discuss deep neural networks. Please check the link of tutorials in the Appendix.

12.5 Pitfalls and Limitations

Machine learning is a powerful technique for healthcare research. From a technical and algorithmic perspective, there are many directions that we can undertake to improve methodology, such as generalizability, less supervision, multimodal training, or learning temporality and irregularity (Xiao et al. 2018).

However, there are some pitfalls and limitations about utilizing machine learning in healthcare that should be considered during model development (Chen et al. 2019). For example, model biases and fairness is a critical issue since the training data we use are usually noisy and biased (Caruana et al. 2015; Ghassemi et al. 2018). We still need human expertise to validate, interpret and adjust the models. Model interpretability is also an important topic from the aspects of (1) human-machine collaboration and (2) building a human-like intelligent machine for medicine (Girkar et al. 2018). Causality is usually not being addressed in most of the clinical machine learning research, yet it is a key feature of clinical decision making. We may need more complicated causal inference algorithms to inform clinical decisions.

We also need to think more about how to deploy the developed machine learning models into clinical workflow. How to utilize them to improve workflow (Horng et al. 2017; Chen et al. 2018), as well as integrate all information acquired by human and machine, to transform them into clinical actions and improve health outcomes are crucial for future clinician-machine collaboration.

12.6 Conclusion

In summary, machine learning is an important and powerful technique for healthcare research. In this chapter, we have shown readers how to reframe a clinical problem into appropriate machine learning tasks, select and employ an algorithm for model training, perform model diagnostics and error analysis, as well as interpret model results. The concepts and tools described in this chapter aim to allow the reader to better understand how to conduct a machine learning project for clinical predictive analytics.

Programming Tutorial Appendix

The tutorials mentioned in this chapter available in the GitHub repository: https://github.com/criticaldata/globalhealthdatabook.git.

References

Abu-Mostafa, Y. S., Lin, H. T., & Magdon-Ismail, M. (2012). Learning from data: A short course. Amlbook.

Bejnordi, B. E., Lin, J., Glass, B., Mullooly, M., Gierach, G. L., Sherman, M. E., et al. (2017) Deep learning-based assessment of tumor-associated stroma for diagnosing breast cancer in histopathology images. In *2017 IEEE 14th international symposium on biomedical imaging (ISBI 2017)* (pp. 929–932). IEEE.

Breiman, L. (2017). *Classification and regression trees*. Routledge.

Breiman, L. (2001). Random forests. *Machine Learning*, *45*(1), 5–32.

Caruana, R., Lou, Y., Gehrke, J., Koch, P., Sturm, M., & Elhadad, N. (2015). Intelligible models for healthcare: Predicting pneumonia risk and hospital 30-day readmission. In *Proceedings of the 21th ACM SIGKDD International Conference on Knowledge Discovery and Data Mining* (pp. 1721–1730). ACM.

Chen, P. C., Gadepalli, K., MacDonald, R., Liu, Y., Nagpal, K., Kohlberger, T., et al. (2018). Microscope 2.0: An augmented reality microscope with real-time artificial intelligence integration, *Nature Medicine*, *25*(9), 1453-1457 arXiv:1812.00825. https://www.nature.com/articles/s41591-019-0539-7

Chen, P. C., Liu, Y., & Peng, L. (2019). How to develop machine learning models for healthcare. *Nature Materials*, *18*(5), 410.

Choi, Y., Chiu, C. Y.-I., & Sontag, D. (2016). Learning low-dimensional representations of medical concepts. *AMIA Summits on Translational Science Proceedings*, *2016*, 41.

Chung, Y.-A., & Weng, W.-H. (2017). Learning deep representations of medical images using Siamese CNNs with application to content-based image retrieval. In *Machine learning for health (ML4H) workshop at NIPS 2017*.

Chung, Y.-A., Weng, W.-H., Tong, S., & Glass, J. (2018). Unsupervised cross-modal alignment of speech and text embedding spaces. In *Advances in neural information processing systems* (pp. 7365–7375).

Chung, Y.-A., Weng, W.-H., Tong, S., & Glass, J. (2019). Towards unsupervised speech-to-text translation. In *2019 IEEE international conference on acoustics, speech and signal processing (ICASSP)* (pp. 7170–7174). IEEE.

Cortes, C., & Vapnik, V. (1995). Support-vector networks. *Machine Learning*, *20*(3), 273–297.

Dernoncourt, F., Lee, J. Y., Uzuner, O., & Szolovits, P. (2017). De-identification of patient notes with recurrent neural networks. *Journal of the American Medical Informatics Association*, *24*(3), 596–606.

Doshi-Velez, F., Ge, Y., & Kohane, I. (2014). Comorbidity clusters in autism spectrum disorders: An electronic health record time-series analysis. *Pediatrics*, *133*(1), e54–e63.

Esteva, A., Kuprel, B., Novoa, R. A., Ko, J., Swetter, S. M., Blau, H. M., et al. (2017). Dermatologist-level classification of skin cancer with deep neural networks. *Nature*, *542*(7639), 115.

Fonarow, G. C., Adams, K. F., Abraham, W. T., Yancy, C. W., Boscardin, W. J., Scientific Advisory Committee, A. D. H. E. R. E., et al. (2005). Risk stratification for in-hospital mortality in acutely decompensated heart failure: Classification and regression tree analysis. *JAMA*, *293*(5), 572–580.

Freund, Y., Schapire, R., & Abe, N. (1999). A short introduction to boosting. *Journal Japanese Society for Artificial Intelligence*, *14*(771–780), 1612.

Friedman, J. H. (2001). Greedy function approximation: A gradient boosting machine. In *Annals of statistics* (pp. 1189–1232).

Gehrmann, S., Dernoncourt, F., Li, Y., Carlson, E. T., Wu, J. T., Welt, J., et al. (2018). Comparing deep learning and concept extraction based methods for patient phenotyping from clinical narratives. *PloS One*, *13*(2), e0192360.

Ghassemi, M., Naumann, T., Doshi-Velez, F., Brimmer, N., Joshi, R., Rumshisky, A., et al. (2014). Unfolding physiological state: Mortality modelling in intensive care units. In *Proceedings of the 20th ACM SIGKDD International Conference on Knowledge Discovery and Data Mining* (pp. 75–84). ACM.

Ghassemi, M., Naumann, T., Schulam, P., Beam, A. L., & Ranganath, R. (2018). Opportunities in machine learning for healthcare. arXiv:1806.00388.

Girkar, U. M., Uchimido, R., Lehman, L.-W. H., Szolovits, P., Celi, L., & Weng, W.-H. (2018). Predicting blood pressure response to fluid bolus therapy using attention-based neural networks for clinical interpretability. In *Machine learning for health (ML4H) workshop at NeurIPS 2018*.

Goodfellow, I., Bengio, Y., & Courville, A. (2016). *Deep learning*. MIT Press.

Gulshan, V., Peng, L., Coram, M., Stumpe, M. C., Derek, W., Narayanaswamy, A., et al. (2016). Development and validation of a deep learning algorithm for detection of diabetic retinopathy in retinal fundus photographs. *JAMA*, *316*(22), 2402–2410.

Henry, J., Pylypchuk, Y., Searcy, T., & Patel, V. (2016). Adoption of electronic health record systems among us non-federal acute care hospitals: 2008–2015. *ONC Data Brief*, *35*, 1–9.

Hinton, G. E., & Salakhutdinov, R. R. (2006). Reducing the dimensionality of data with neural networks. *Science*, *313*(5786), 504–507.

Hoerl, A. E., & Kennard, R. W. (1970). Ridge regression: Biased estimation for nonorthogonal problems. *Technometrics*, *12*(1), 55–67.

Horng, S., Sontag, D. A., Halpern, Y., Jernite, Y., Shapiro, N. I., & Nathanson, L. A. (2017). Creating an automated trigger for sepsis clinical decision support at emergency department triage using machine learning. *PloS One*, *12*(4), e0174708.

Hsu, T.-M. H., Weng, W.-H., Boag, W., McDermott, M., & Szolovits, P. (2018). Unsupervised multimodal representation learning across medical images and reports. In *Machine learning for health (ML4H) workshop at NeurIPS 2018*.

Jolliffe, I. (2011). *Principal component analysis*. Springer.

Komorowski, M., Celi, L. A., Badawi, O., Gordon, A. C., & Faisal, A. A. (2018). The artificial intelligence clinician learns optimal treatment strategies for sepsis in intensive care. *Nature Medicine*, *24*(11), 1716.

Krizhevsky, A., Sutskever, I., & Hinton, G. E. (2012). Imagenet classification with deep convolutional neural networks. In *Advances in neural information processing systems* (pp. 1097–1105).

Lehman, E. P., Krishnan, R. G., Zhao, X., Mark, R. G., & Lehman, L.-W. H. (2018). Representation learning approaches to detect false arrhythmia alarms from ECG dynamics. In *Machine learning for healthcare conference* (pp. 571–586).

Liu, Y., Gadepalli, K., Norouzi, M., Dahl, G. E., Kohlberger, T., Boyko, A., et al. (2017). Detecting cancer metastases on gigapixel pathology images. arXiv:1703.02442.

Liu, G., Hsu, T.-M, H., McDermott, M., Boag, W., Weng, W.-H., Szolovits, P., et al. (2019). Clinically accurate chest x-ray report generation. In *Machine Learning for Healthcare* arXiv:1904.02633.

Nagpal, K., Foote, D., Liu, Y., Wulczyn, E., Tan, F., Olson, N., et al. (2019). Development and validation of a deep learning algorithm for improving gleason scoring of prostate cancer. *NPJ digital medicine*, 2(1), 1-10. arXiv:1811.06497. https://www.nature.com/articles/s41746-019-0112-2

Pivovarov, R., Perotte, A. J., Grave, E., Angiolillo, J., Wiggins, C. H., & Elhadad, N. (2015). Learning probabilistic phenotypes from heterogeneous EHR data. *Journal of Biomedical Informatics*, *58*, 156–165.

Raghu, A., Komorowski, M., Celi, L. A., Szolovits, P., & Ghassemi, M. (2017). Machine Learning for Healthcare: Continuous state-space models for optimal sepsis treatment-a deep reinforcement learning approach.

Rumelhart, D. E., Hinton, G. E., Williams, R. J., et al. (1988). Learning representations by back-propagating errors. *Cognitive Modeling*, *5*(3), 1.

Silver, D., Huang, A., Maddison, C. J., Guez, A., Sifre, L., Van Den Driessche, G., et al. (2016). Mastering the game of go with deep neural networks and tree search. *Nature*, *529*(7587), 484.

Tibshirani, R. (1996). Regression shrinkage and selection via the lasso. *Journal of the Royal Statistical Society: Series B (Methodological)*, *58*(1), 267–288.

van der Maaten, L., & Hinton, G. (2008). Visualizing data using t-SNE. *Journal of Machine Learning Research*, *9*, 2579–2605.

Wei-Weng, H., & Szolovits, P. (2018). Mapping unparalleled clinical professional and consumer languages with embedding alignment. In *2018 KDD workshop on machine learning for medicine and healthcare*.

Weng, W.-H., Chung, Y.-A., & Szolovits, P. (2019). Unsupervised clinical language translation. In *25th ACM SIGKDD conference on knowledge discovery and data mining (KDD 2019)*.

Weng, W.-H., Gao, M., He, Z., Yan, S., & Szolovits, P. (2017). Representation and reinforcement learning for personalized glycemic control in septic patients. In *Machine learning for health (ML4H) workshop at NIPS 2017*.

Weng, W.-H., Wagholikar, K. B., McCray, A. T., Szolovits, P., & Chueh, H. C. (2017). Medical subdomain classification of clinical notes using a machine learning-based natural language processing approach. *BMC Medical Informatics and Decision Making*, *17*(1), 155.

Wu, Y., Schuster, M., Chen, Z., Le, Q. V., Norouzi, M., Macherey, W., et al. (2016). Google's neural machine translation system: Bridging the gap between human and machine translation. arXiv:1609.08144.

Xiao, C., Choi, E., & Sun, J. (2018). Opportunities and challenges in developing deep learning models using electronic health records data: A systematic review. *Journal of the American Medical Informatics Association*, *25*(10), 1419–1428.

Yala, A., Barzilay, R., Salama, L., Griffin, M., Sollender, G., Bardia, A., et al. (2017). Using machine learning to parse breast pathology reports. *Breast Cancer Research and Treatment*, *161*(2), 203–211.

Zou, H., & Hastie, T. (2005) elasticnet: Elastic net regularization and variable selection. In *R package version* (p. 1).

13

Modeling and Prediction Tools: Random Forest and Support Vector Machines

Siqi Liu, Hao Du, and Mengling Feng

Abstract In this chapter, we aim to explain the principles that make random forest (RF) and support vector machines (SVMs) successful modelling and prediction tools for a variety of applications. We try to achieve this by presenting the basic ideas of RF and SVMs, together with an illustrative example using the MIMIC III database. The advantages and limitations of both methods are discussed in the chapter. The chapter provides some guidance for choosing a machine learning model, building and training the model, validating model performance and interpreting the results with the Python programming language.

Keywords Predictive model · Mortality prediction · Random forest · Support vector machine

Learning Objectives

- To understand the basic ideas of random forest and support vector machine
- To understand the advantages and limitations while choosing a machine learning model
- To build and evaluate a machine learning model on ICU mortality prediction problem
- To interpret the model results in clinical problems

13.1 Background

In this chapter, we are going to introduce two commonly used statistical models for healthcare data: random forest and support vector machines (SVM). These two models are mainly used for two purposes: first, to create robust and accurate predictive models and second, these models are used in order to evaluate and interpret the

S. Liu · H. Du · M. Feng (✉)
Saw Swee Hock School of Public Health, National University of Singapore and National University Health System,
10-01 Science Drive 2, Singapore, Singapore
e-mail: ephfm@nus.edu.sg

features (clinical variables). To their advantage, these methods both prevent overfitting and obtain reliable results. Additionally, random forest reduces bias by utilizing average ensemble and SVM uses kerneling to introduce non-linearity. More details will be explained in the following chapter.

In the following chapter and exercises, we are going to explain and demonstrate how these two models work and how to use them.

13.2 Random Forest

Random forest is an ensemble model which fits multiple decision tree classifiers on subsets of the training data and uses averaging to improve the predictive score and control over-fitting (Liaw and Wiener 2002). To understand a random forest, we must start with the basic building block of the model: the decision tree model.

13.2.1 Decision Tree

A decision tree model is a supervised model that learns to predict the expected output by answering a series of questions and making decisions based on the answers (Safavian and Landgrebe 1991). The concept of a decision tree model is subconsciously used by us throughout our daily life. For example, clinicians may intuitively evaluate a patient's condition by asking a series of questions, progressively reaching a diagnostic conclusion. We will use a clinical example to illustrate this concept further: predicting a patient's ICU mortality from first day ICU admission data.

In order to predict ICU mortality, we need to work through a series of queries. We may begin with a reasonable initial question given the domain knowledge, such as asking how old the patient is. In general, the survival rate of a young patient will be higher than the elderly in ICU. After this question, we will look at other predictive variables that could be helpful in determining a patient's ICU mortality, such as the gender of the patient, laboratory results (particularly abnormal values), and treatments the patient may be receiving. By asking these questions, ICU clinicians may garner the likelihood that the patient might survive their ICU stay. A decision tree model would similarly follow that clinical thinking process. It designs a set of questions that segregates the data with each subsequent question, narrowing our possible values until we are confident enough to make a single prediction. This example clinical decision tree is illustrated in Diagram 13.1. The complexity of a decision tree can be represented by tree depth, the number of steps from the root node to the leaf node. In Diagram 13.1, the depth of the decision tree is three. In practical analysis, if the depth is too large, then your model is too complex and you might face an overfitting problem. If the depth is too small, then your model might not capture the variance in data and thus might underfit the problem.

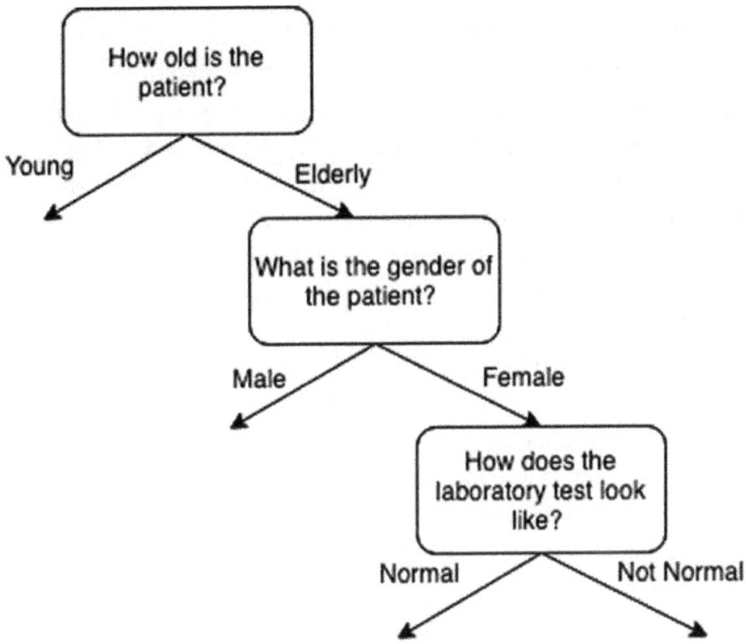

Diagram 13.1 Clinical decision tree

In brief, that is the high-level concept of a decision tree: a flowchart of questions leading to a prediction. Now, we take the mighty leap from a single decision tree to a random forest.

13.2.2 From Decision Tree to Random Forest

Health care is incredibly complex and there are many factors to take into account when clinicians try to make a prediction. Furthermore, every clinician approaches a problem with different background knowledge. Even if they are encountering the same patient, decisions and treatments from any two clinicians may differ from each other. This challenge is similar for decision tree models: if looking at different sub-samples of training data, decision models may fit them with different flowcharts of questions and get different conclusions. In technical terms, there exists variance in predictions because they are widely spread around the correct answer. If we collect a group of hundreds or thousands of clinicians, some making the correct prediction and some of making incorrect predictions, we might assume the majority represents best practice and thus take the most popular prediction as the final decision. This is the concept of a random forest. The fundamental idea is to ensemble many decision trees into a single model to reduce the prediction variance. Individually, the prediction from a single human or decision tree may not be accurate, but by combining multiple observations, the variance is reduced and the predictions are more likely aggregated around the true outcome.

In a random forest model, each decision tree only accesses a random subset of training data. This increases the diversity of the ensemble model, thus improving the robustness of the overall model. That is why we call this model "random." When the model makes a prediction, random forest takes outputs from all individual decision tree models and outputs the prediction with the highest votes among the individual models. In our example here, the ICU mortality prediction is a classification task, where we are predicting a binary outcome of mortality (Death/Survival). In other cases where the targets are a continuous value (such as "ICU Free Days"), we would use a regression analysis and would take the average for the predicted values.

Since we are looking at a binary supervised classification problem in our example (ICU mortality), we may also consider another popular statistical method to model the data: a support vector machine (SVM).

13.3 Support Vector Machines (SVM)

A support vector machine (SVM) is a supervised machine learning algorithm that is used for both classification and regression purposes (Hearst et al. 1998). That said, SVMs are more commonly employed for classification problems, so we will be focusing on SVM with classification problems here.

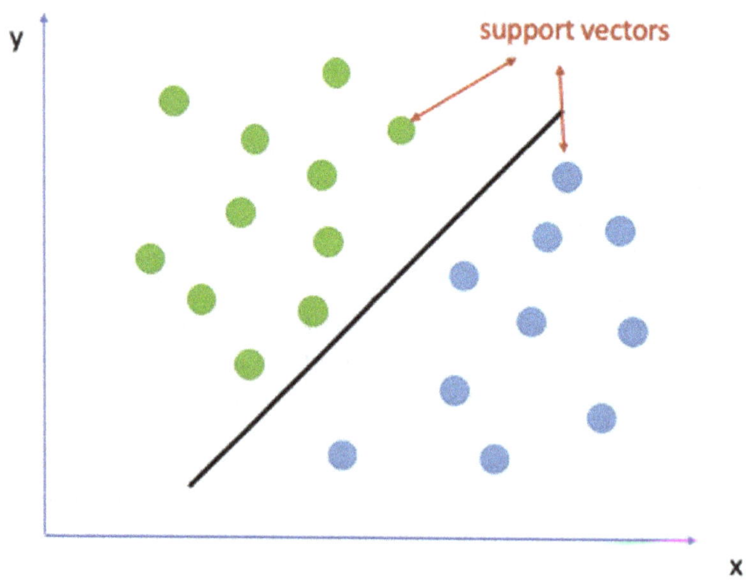

Fig. 13.1 SVM and support vectors

The concept of an SVM is finding a dividing plane that maximizes the margin between two classes in a dataset and achieves the best fit, as illustrated in Fig. 13.1. This plane is called a hyperplane.

Support vectors are the points nearest to the hyperplane. If these points are removed, the position of hyperplane would likely be altered to divide the dataset better. In other words, support vectors are the data points (vectors) that define the hyperplane. Therefore, they are considered to be the critical elements of the dataset.

13.3.1 What is a Hyperplane?

As shown in Fig. 13.1, there are two features for the classification task. The data are in a two-dimensional space, so we can think of a hyperplane as a straight line which classifies the data into two subsets. Intuitively, the farther the data points (support vectors) lie from the hyperplane, the more confident we are that they have been correctly classified. Therefore, the model will place the data points as far away as possible from the hyperplane while making sure the data points are correctly classified. When we feed new data to the SVM model, whatever side of the hyperplane it falls determines the class that it is assigned.

13.3.2 How Can We Identify the Right Hyperplane?

The hyperplane is determined by the maximum margin, which is the distance between a hyperplane and the nearest data point from either class. The goal of fitting an SVM model is to choose a hyperplane with the highest possible margin between the hyperplane and any training data points, which grants the best chance for new data to be classified correctly. We will now illustrate some scenarios on how an SVM model can fit the data and identify the right hyperplane.

Scenario 1 (Fig. 13.2): Here, we have three hyperplanes (A, B and C). In identifying the best hyperplane to classify blue dots and green dots, "hyperplane "B" has clearly best performed the segregation of the two classes in this scenario.

Scenario 2 (Fig. 13.3): If all three hyperplanes (A, B, C) has segregated the classes well, then the best hyperplane will be the one that maximizes the linear distances (margins) between nearest data point for either of the classes. In this scenario, the margin for hyperplane B is higher when compared to both A and C. Hence, we determine the best hyperplane as B. The intuition behind this is that a hyperplane with more considerable margins is more robust; if we select a hyperplane having low margin then there is a higher chance of misclassification.

Scenario 3 (Fig. 13.4): In this scenario, we cannot create a linear hyperplane between the two classes. This is where it can get tricky. Data is rarely ever as clean as our simple examples above. A dataset will often look more like the mixture of dots below - representing a non-linearly separable dataset.

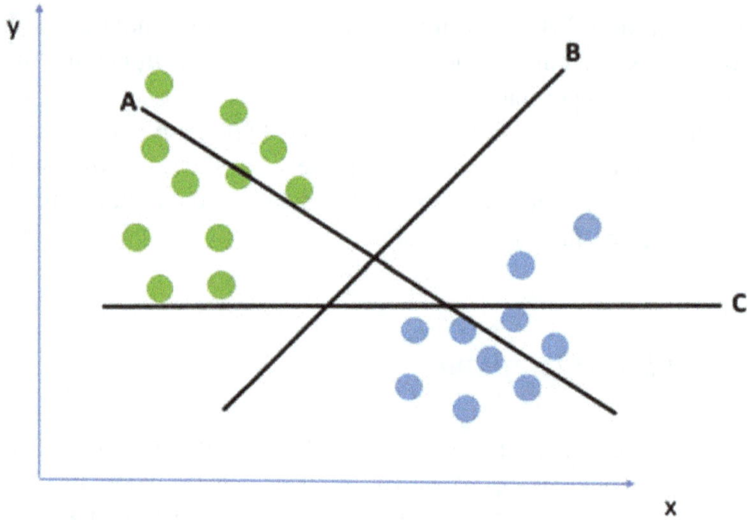

Fig. 13.2 Hyperplane identification, scenario 1

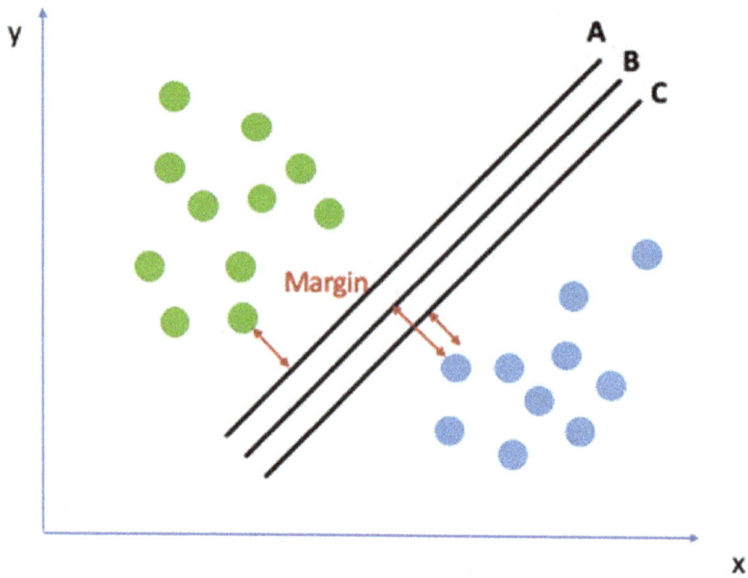

Fig. 13.3 Hyperplane identification, scenario 2

So how can a SVM classify these two classes? With datasets like this, it is sometimes necessary to move away from a 2-dimensional (2-D) view of the data to a 3-D view. Imagine that our two sets of coloured dots above are sitting on a sheet and this sheet is lifted suddenly, launching the dots into the air. While the dots are up in the air, you use the sheet to separate them. This 'lifting' of the dots represents the mapping of data into a higher dimension. This is known as kernelling (Fig. 13.5).

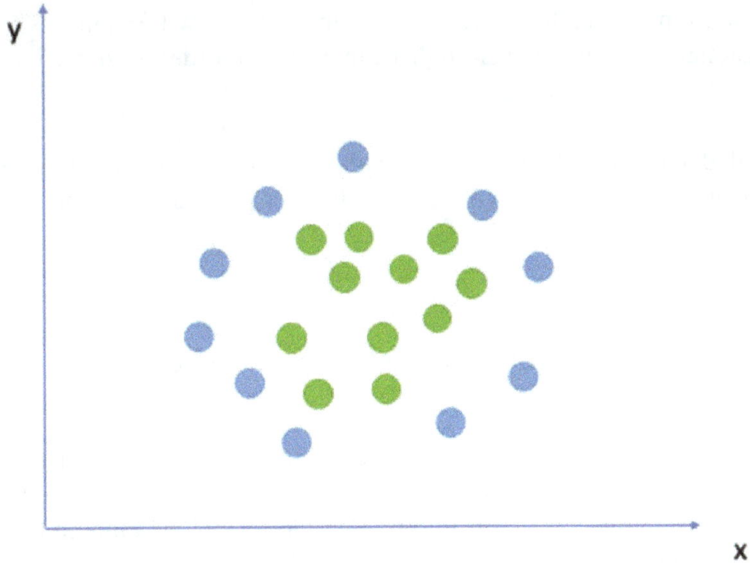

Fig. 13.4 Hyperplane identification, scenario 3

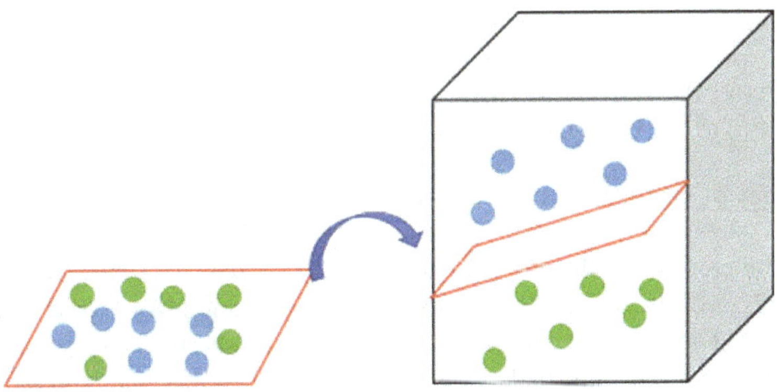

Fig. 13.5 Hyperplane identification, kernelling

Kernelling uses functions to take low dimensional input space and transform it into a higher dimensional space. For example, it converts a non-separable problem into a separable problem for classification. In Fig. 13.4, the kernels map the 2-D data into 3-D space. In the 2-D space, it is impossible to separate blue and green dots with linear functions. After the kernel transformation maps them to 3-D space, the blue and green dots can be separated using a hyperplane. The most commonly used kernels are "linear" kernel, "radial basis function" (RBF) kernel, "polynomial" kernel and others (Hsu et al. 2003). Among them, RBF kernel is the most useful in non-linear separation problems.

In real life scenarios, the dimension of the data can be far higher than 3-D. For instance, we want to use a patient's demographics and lab values to predict the ICU mortality, the number of available predictive variables is easily as high as 10+

dimensions. In this case, the kernel we used in the SVM will require us to map the 10-dimensional data into an even higher dimension in order to identify an optimal hyperplane.

We will demonstrate how to analyse this problem with the above statistical methods using Jupyter Notebook and the Python programming language in the following exercises.

13.4 Limitations of Random Forest and SVM

There are limitations in utilizing random forest for healthcare data. First, these models are sometimes difficult to interpret. For random forest, we may be able to interpret individual decision trees; however interpreting the ensembled random forest model is difficult for complex healthcare data. For SVMs the results are also difficult to interpret due to kernel transformations. Secondly, in tuning the model, some hyper-parameters of these methods need to be determined by users and cannot be optimized.

13.5 Exercise Introduction

In this series of exercises, we will begin to apply statistical learning methods such as random forest and support vector machines (SVM) on real world clinical electronic health records (EHR) data. We are going to use data extracted from a publicly available research clinical dataset, the **M**edical **I**nformation **M**art for **I**ntensive **C**are (MIMIC III). The database contains granular, deidentified ICU data generated from over 70 intensive care unit beds with medical, surgical, cardiac, and neurological patients. Data in MIMIC-III includes demographic information, vital signs, medication records, laboratory measurements, observations, fluid balance, procedure codes, diagnostic codes, imaging reports, hospital length of stay, survival data, and so on.

13.5.1 Jupyter Notebook

Jupyter Notebook is a web application that creates an interactive environment for you to code and view the outputs of your results. It is widely used in data cleaning and transformation, statistical modelling, data visualization, machine learning, etc. Instructions for Jupyter Notebook installation can be found at: http://jupyter.org/install.html. We will be using the Python3 kernel of Jupyter Notebook in this series of exercises.

13.5.2 Data

In this example, the problem we will investigate is prediction of ICU mortality using patient demographics and first laboratory tests. We have the demographic information and first laboratory measurements for patients admitted to the ICU. These information reflect the patient state at the moment they were admitted to ICU and we are going to use them to estimate the probability that the patient is going to survive in ICU. In statistical modeling or machine learning, this is a supervised classification problem. It is a supervised problem because, besides features (demographics and first lab measurements), we also have labels (ICU mortality) for model training. The trained model would be able to classify the patient's condition into ICU survival group or ICU non-survival group, thus making it a classification problem.

13.5.3 Workflow

After the clinical question is defined, we will follow a workflow to analyze and answer the question. The workflow is as follows:

1. Problem statement and data specification
2. Identification and extraction of the required data
3. Data cleaning and missing value processing
4. Data formatting and preparation for modelling
5. Model training
6. Model performance evaluation
7. Parameter adjustment and fine-tuning
8. Model interpretation and report

Our clinical question has been defined above, so we will start from step 2 in exercise 1. These exercises can be found online at: https://github.com/criticaldata/globalhealthdatabook.

References

Hearst, M. A., Dumais, S. T., Osuna, E., Platt, J., & Scholkopf, B. (1998). Support vector machines. *IEEE Intelligent Systems and their Applications, 13*(4), 18–28.

Hsu, C. W., Chang, C. C., & Lin, C. J. (2003). A practical guide to support vector classification.

Liaw, A., & Wiener, M. (2002). Classification and regression by random forest. *R News, 2*(3), 18–22.

Safavian, S. R., & Landgrebe, D. (1991). A survey of decision tree classifier methodology. *IEEE Transactions on Systems, Man, and Cybernetics, 21*(3), 660–674.

Permissions

All chapters in this book were first published by Springer; hereby published with permission under the Creative Commons Attribution License or equivalent. Every chapter published in this book has been scrutinized by our experts. Their significance has been extensively debated. The topics covered herein carry significant information for a comprehensive understanding. They may even be implemented as practical applications or may be referred to as a beginning point for further studies.

The contributors of this book come from diverse backgrounds, making this book a truly international effort. We would like to thank all the contributing authors for lending their expertise to make the book truly unique. They have played a crucial role in the development of this book. Without their invaluable contributions this book wouldn't have been possible. They have made vital efforts to compile up to date information on the varied aspects of this subject to make this book a valuable addition to the collection of many professionals and students.

This book was conceptualized with the vision of imparting up-to-date and integrated information in this field. To ensure the same, a matchless editorial board was set up. Every individual on the board went through rigorous rounds of assessment to prove their worth. After which they invested a large part of their time researching and compiling the most relevant data for our readers.

The editorial board has been involved in producing this book since its inception. They have spent rigorous hours researching and exploring the diverse topics which have resulted in the successful publishing of this book. They have passed on their knowledge of decades through this book. To expedite this challenging task, the publisher supported the team at every step. A small team of assistant editors was also appointed to further simplify the editing procedure and attain best results for the readers.

Apart from the editorial board, the designing team has also invested a significant amount of their time in understanding the subject and creating the most relevant covers. They scrutinized every image to scout for the most suitable representation of the subject and create an appropriate cover for the book.

The publishing team has been an ardent support to the editorial, designing and production team. Their endless efforts to recruit the best for this project, has resulted in the accomplishment of this book. They are a veteran in the field of academics and their pool of knowledge is as vast as their experience in printing. Their expertise and guidance has proved useful at every step. Their uncompromising quality standards have made this book an exceptional effort. Their encouragement from time to time has been an inspiration for everyone.

The publisher and the editorial board hope that this book will prove to be a valuable piece of knowledge for students, practitioners and scholars across the globe.

Index

A
Agile Software Development, 33-34, 37, 51
Approval Rate, 84-85
Artificial Intelligence, 3-4, 6, 10-11, 14-15, 61, 63, 190-191, 206-207
Auxiliary Variables, 79-81, 87, 90

B
Blockchain Technology, 9, 14, 94, 102
Bootstrapping, 89, 92-93

C
Causal Loop Diagrams, 73-74, 76, 85, 93
Clinical Decision Support, 5, 7, 10, 13-14, 207
Clinical Prediction, 105-106, 190-192, 200, 204
Clustering, 121-123, 136, 141-144, 146-147, 149, 151-152, 157-161, 167, 188, 196, 200, 203, 205
Collaboration, 3, 8-9, 11-13, 56, 65, 67-68, 74, 205
Coordination, 74, 95, 102
Crash Course, 105-106, 108
Cross-Validation, 105, 115-116, 118, 120, 187, 197
Cryptography, 60, 94, 102

D
Data Mapping, 53, 59
Data Models, 54, 56, 58
Data Pipeline, 53, 60
Data-Rich Ecosystems, 73-75, 82, 91
Databases, 53-57, 61, 65, 67-68, 99, 127
Decision Tree, 111, 113, 121, 174-175, 179, 187, 190, 201, 210-212, 217
Deidentification, 53, 200
Design Thinking, 16-22, 24, 26, 30-35, 51
Desirability, 16, 19-20, 49
Dimensionality Reduction, 139, 188, 200, 203-204
Disease Repositories, 53-54

E
Electronic Health Records, 3-4, 6, 14-15, 53, 56, 123, 189, 208, 216
Epidemiology, 72, 76, 84
Equilibrium, 77, 79, 86
Error Analysis, 89, 199, 205

F
Feedback Loops, 73, 77-78, 83, 85
Frail Individuals, 25, 44
Full Recovery, 29
Funding Announcement, 68-69, 71
Funding Proposal, 63-66, 70-71
Funding Sources, 63, 67, 70-72
Funding Strategy, 63, 67, 70-71

G
Gini Index, 112-113, 120, 175, 201
Global Health, 3-4, 8-14, 16-17, 19-21, 30, 32-37, 39, 43, 49-52, 63, 73-74, 82-85, 91, 93
Grant Writing, 63, 70-72

H
Health Information Exchange, 3-4, 6, 8, 13-15, 101
Health Information Technology, 3-4, 6, 15
Health Outcome, 40
Healthcare Systems, 3-4, 11, 17, 73
Homologation, 59-60
Hyperplane, 114-116, 118, 202, 213-216
Hypotheses, 36, 41

I
Ideation, 16, 27-28, 35, 37
Implementation Research, 63-64, 72
Indentation, 108
Information Technology, 3-6, 13, 15
Innovation, 13, 16-20, 22-24, 27-37, 39, 41-43, 46-47, 50-52, 63-65, 67-69, 72, 74, 84
Innovation Workshop, 33, 39, 42
Intellectual Property, 67, 84
Interoperability, 9, 12, 14, 74, 84, 91, 94

K
Kernel Function, 115-116, 119

L
Loss Function, 110, 190, 194

Lotka-Volterra Model, 80-81

M
Machine Learning, 6, 10-11, 14-15, 54-55, 61, 82, 91, 93, 105-107, 110, 112, 119-124, 140, 143, 158, 161, 163, 178, 189-192, 194-197, 200, 202-203, 205-209, 212, 216-217

Mean Squared Error, 110-111

Model Fit, 105, 110

Mortality Prediction, 161, 193, 209, 212

N
Negative Polarity, 77, 86-87

Node Purity, 112-113

O
Opportunity Score, 47

Outcome Driven Innovation, 33-35, 41, 46

Outcome Map, 43-44, 47, 49-50

P
Parameterization, 82, 92

Pharmaceutical Companies, 40, 86

Point of View, 27

Policy Interventions, 79-80

Positive Polarity, 77

Principal Component Analysis, 139, 204, 207

Probabilistic Methods, 82, 91

Product Development, 23, 33-34, 37-38, 41, 43, 45, 48-50, 76

Product Lifecycle, 33, 38, 42

Prototype, 26-27, 29, 33, 49, 51, 60

Python, 82, 93, 105-109, 120-122, 124, 134, 140, 143, 161, 164, 188-189, 203-204, 209, 216

Q
Quality of Life, 25

R
Radial Basis Function, 115-116, 202, 215

Random Forest, 105, 111-113, 116, 119-123, 161, 180, 189, 201, 204, 209-212, 216-217

Recursive Binary Splitting, 112-113, 175

Research Proposal, 63, 65-66, 71-72

S
Scalability, 6, 98, 100

Statistical Learning, 73, 82, 121, 180, 189, 203, 216

Stock And Flow Diagrams, 73, 76, 79-80, 82

Support Vector Machine, 105, 113, 119, 121, 190, 194, 202, 209, 212

Support Vectors, 114, 212-213

System Dynamics, 73-76, 79-82, 86, 89-93

T
Technical Feasibility, 43, 49

V
Viability, 19, 50

W
Workforce Capacity, 4, 74

www.ingramcontent.com/pod-product-compliance
Lightning Source LLC
LaVergne TN
LVHW062237200926
848484LV00006B/1558